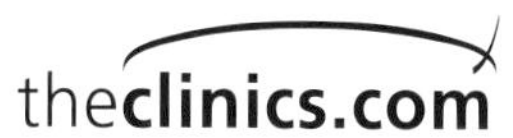

MEDICAL CLINICS
OF NORTH AMERICA

Minority Health and Disparities-Related Issues: Part II

GUEST EDITORS
Eddie L. Greene, MD
Charles R. Thomas, Jr., MD

September 2005 • Volume 89 • Number 5

SAUNDERS

An Imprint of Elsevier, Inc.
PHILADELPHIA LONDON TORONTO MONTREAL SYDNEY TOKYO

W.B. SAUNDERS COMPANY
A Division of Elsevier Inc.

1600 John F. Kennedy Boulevard • Suite 1800 • Philadelphia, Pennsylvania 19103-2899

http://www.theclinics.com

MEDICAL CLINICS OF NORTH AMERICA   **Volume 89, Number 5**
September 2005   **ISSN 0025-7125**
Editor: Heather Cullen   **ISBN 1-4160-2726-2**

The ideas and opinions expressed in *Medical Clinics of North America* do not necessarily reflect those of the Publisher. The Publisher does not assume any responsibility for any injury and/or damage to persons or property arising out of or related to any use of the material contained in this periodical. The reader is advised to check the appropriate medical literature and the product information currently provided by the manufacturer of each drug to be administered to verify the dosage, the method and duration of administration, or contraindications. It is the responsibility of the treating physician or other health care professional, relying on independent experience and knowledge of the patient, to determine drug dosages and the best treatment for the patient. Mention of any product in this issue should not be construed as endorsement by the contributors, editors, or the Publisher of the product or manufacturers' claims.

Medical Clinics of North America (ISSN 0025-7125) is published bimonthly by Elsevier. Corporate and editorial offices: 1600 John F. Kennedy Boulevard, Suite 1800, Philadelphia, PA 19103-2899. Accounting and circulation offices: 6277 Sea Harbor Drive, Orlando, FL 32887-4800. Periodicals postage paid at Orlando, FL 32862, and additional mailing offices. Subscription prices are USD 140 per year for US individuals, USD 244 per year for US institutions, USD 70 per year for US students, USD 180 per year for Canadian individuals, USD 311 per year for Canadian institutions, USD 205 per year for international individuals, USD 311 per year for international institutions and USD 103 per year for Canadian and foreign students/residents. To receive student/resident rate, orders must be accompanied by name of affiliated institution, date of term, and the *signature* of program/residency coordinator on institution letterhead. Orders will be billed at individual rate until proof of status is received. Foreign air speed delivery is included in all *Clinics* subscription prices. All prices are subject to change without notice. POSTMASTER: Send address changes to *Medical Clinics of North America*, W.B. Saunders Company, Periodicals Fulfillment, Orlando, FL 32887-4800. **Customer Service: 1-800-654-2452 (US). From outside of the USA, call (+1) 407-345-1000. E-mail: hhspcs@harcourt.com.**

Reprints. For copies of 100 or more, of articles in this publication, please contact the Commercial Reprints Department, Elsevier Inc., 360 Park Avenue South, New York, New York 10010-1710. Tel.: (+1) (212) 633-3813; Fax: (+1) (212) 462-1935; E-mail: reprints@elsevier.com.

Medical Clinics of North America is also published in Spanish by McGraw-Hill Interamericana Editores S. A., P.O. Box 5-237, 06500 Mexico, D.F., Mexico.

Medical Clinics of North America is covered in *Index Medicus, Current Contents, ASCA, Excerpta Medica, Science Citation Index,* and *ISI/BIOMED.*

Printed in the United States of America.

GOAL STATEMENT

The goal of *Medical Clinics of North America* is to keep practicing physicians up to date with current clinical practice by providing timely articles reviewing the state of the art in patient care.

ACCREDITATION

The *Medical Clinics of North America* is planned and implemented in accordance with the Essential Areas and Policies of the Accreditation Council for Continuing Medical Education (ACCME) through the joint sponsorship of the University of Virginia School of Medicine and Elsevier. The University of Virginia School of Medicine is accredited by the ACCME to provide continuing medical education for physicians.

The University of Virginia School of Medicine designates this educational activity for a maximum of 90 category 1 credits per year, 15 category 1 credits per issue, toward the AMA Physician's Recognition Award. Each physician should claim only those credits that he/she actually spent in the activity.

The American Medical Association has determined that physicians not licensed in the US who participate in this CME activity are eligible for AMA PRA category 1 credit.

Category 1 credit can be earned by reading the text material, taking the CME examination online at *http://www.theclinics.com/home/cme*, and completing the evaluation. Each test question must be answered correctly; you will have the opportunity to retake any questions answered incorrectly. Following successful completion of the test and the evaluation, you may print your certificate.

FACULTY DISCLOSURE

As a provider accredited by the Accreditation Council for Continuing Medical Education (ACCME), the Office of Continuing Medical Education of the University of Virginia School of Medicine must ensure balance, independence, objectivity, and scientific rigor in all its individually sponsored or jointly sponsored educational activities. All authors/editors participating in a sponsored activity are expected to disclose to the readers any significant financial interest or other relationship (1) with the manufacturer(s) of any commercial product(s) and/or provider(s) of commercial services discussed in an educational presentation and (2) with any commercial supporters of the activity (significant financial interest or other relationship can include such things as grants or research support, employee, consultant, stock holder, member of speakers bureau, etc.) The intent of this disclosure is not to prevent authors/editors with a significant financial or other relationship from writing an article, but rather to provide readers with information on which they can make their own judgments. It remains for the readers to determine whether the author's/editor's interest or relationships may influence the article with regard to exposition or conclusion.

The authors/editors listed below have identified no professional or financial affiliations related to their publication:

David C. Chang, PhD, MPH, MBA; Luther T. Clark, MD; Edward E. Cornwell, MD; Heather Cullen, Acquisitions Editor; Wade Douglas, MD; Leonard E. Egede, MD, MS; Crystal A. Gadegbeku, MD; Eddie L. Greene, MD; Michael L. Hicks, MD; Wesley L. Hicks, Jr., MD; Kenneth A. Jamerson, MD; Janice P. Lea, MD; Pablo Mojica-Manosa, MD; Groesbeck P. Parham, MD; Nestor R. Rigual, MD; Sharon Spencer, MD; Charles R. Thomas, Jr., MD; Cheryl L. Walker, MD; and, Carlton J. Young, MD.

The authors listed below have identified the following professional or financial affiliations related to their publication:

Samuel Dagogo-Jack, MD, FRCP is a consultant for GlaxoSmithKline, Eli Lily, Aventis, and has received grants/research support for Pfizer and Novartis.

Clifton Kew, MD has received research support via grants from Astellas Pharmaceuticals, Novartis Pharmaceuticals.

Edith P. Mitchell, MD, FACP is on the speakers' bureau and has received research support for Sanofi, Pfizer, Bristol-Myers Squibb, Genentech and Roche.

Disclosure of discussion of non-FDA approved uses for pharmaceutical products and/or medical devices: The University of Virginia School of Medicine, as an ACCME provider, requires that all authors/editors identify and disclose any "off label" uses for pharmaceutical products and/or for medical devices. The University of Virginia School of Medicine recommends that each reader fully review all the available data on new products or procedures prior to instituting them with patients.

All authors who provided disclosures will not be discussing any off-label uses.

The following authors have not provided disclosure of off-label information.

Billy R. Ballard, MD; L.D. Britt, MD, MPH, FACS, FCCM.

TO ENROLL

To enroll in the Medical Clinics of North America Continuing Medical Education program, call customer service at 1-800-654-2452 or sign up online at *http://www.theclinics.com/home/cme*. The CME program is available to subscribers for an additional annual fee of USD 195.

FORTHCOMING ISSUES

November 2005

Medical Toxicology
Christopher P. Holstege, MD, and
Daniel E. Rusyniak, MD, *Guest Editors*

January 2006

Allergy
Anthony Montanaro, MD, *Guest Editor*

RECENT ISSUES

July 2005

**Minority Health and Disparities-Related Issues:
Part I**
Eddie L. Greene, MD, and
Charles R. Thomas, Jr., MD, *Guest Editors*

May 2005

Chronic Kidney Disease
Ajay K. Singh, MB, MRCP(UK), *Guest Editor*

March 2005

**Screening, Prevention, and Treatment of
Esophageal, Gastric, and Hepatic Malignancies**
Mitchell S. Cappell, MD, PhD, FACG, *Guest Editor*

THE CLINICS ARE NOW AVAILABLE ONLINE!

Access your subscription at:
http://www.theclinics.com

GUEST EDITORS

EDDIE L. GREENE, MD, Associate Professor (Medicine), Division of Nephrology, Department of Internal Medicine, Mayo Clinic College of Medicine, Rochester, Minnesota

CHARLES R. THOMAS, JR., MD, Professor and Vice Chairman, Department of Radiation Oncology; and Professor (Medical Oncology), San Antonio Cancer Institute, University of Texas Health Science Center at San Antonio, San Antonio, Texas

CONTRIBUTORS

BILLY R. BALLARD, MD, Chairman, Department of Pathology, Anatomy and Cell Biology, Meharry Medical College, Nashville, Tennessee

L.D. BRITT, MD, MPH, FACS, FCCM, Department of Surgery, Eastern Virginia Medical School, Norfolk, Virginia

DAVID C. CHANG, PhD, MPH, MBA, Department of Surgery, Johns Hopkins School of Medicine, Baltimore, Maryland

LUTHER T. CLARK, MD, Professor (Clinical Medicine); and Chief, Division of Cardiovascular Medicine, Department of Medicine, State University of New York Downstate Medical Center, Brooklyn, New York

EDWARD E. CORNWELL, MD, Department of Surgery, Johns Hopkins School of Medicine, Baltimore, Maryland

SAMUEL DAGOGO-JACK, MD, FRCP, Professor (Medicine, Endocrinology, Diabetes, and Metabolism), Division of Endocrinology, Diabetes, and Metabolism, Department of Medicine, University of Tennessee Health Sciences Center, Memphis, Tennessee

WADE DOUGLAS, MD, Fellow, Department of Head and Neck Surgery, Roswell Park Cancer Institute, Buffalo, New York

LEONARD E. EGEDE, MD, MS, Assistant Professor (Medicine), Division of General Internal Medicine, Department of Medicine, Medical University of South Carolina; Director, Charleston Veterans Affairs Target Research Enhancement Program; and Staff Physician, Ralph H. Johnson Veterans Affairs Medical Center, Charleston, South Carolina

CRYSTAL A. GADEGBEKU, MD, Assistant Professor, Division of Nephrology, Department of Internal Medicine, University of Michigan Health System, Ann Arbor, Michigan

MICHAEL L. HICKS, MD, Director, Gynecologic Oncology, Michigan Cancer Institute, Pontiac, Michigan

WESLEY L. HICKS, JR, MD, Attending Surgeon and Associate Professor (Otolaryngology/ Head and Neck Surgery), Department of Head and Neck Surgery, Roswell Park Cancer Institute, Buffalo, New York

KENNETH A. JAMERSON, MD, Professor, Division of Nephrology, Department of Internal Medicine, University of Michigan Health System, Ann Arbor, Michigan

CLIFTON KEW, MD, Assistant Professor (Medicine and Surgery), Division of Nephrology, Department of Medicine, University of Alabama at Birmingham, Birmingham, Alabama

JANICE P. LEA, MD, Associate Professor, Renal Division, Department of Medicine, Emory University School of Medicine, Atlanta, Georgia

EDITH P. MITCHELL, MD, FACP, Clinical Professor (Medicine), Division of Medical Oncology, Kimmerl Cancer Center, Thomas Jefferson University, Philadelphia, Pennsylvania

PABLO MOJICA-MANOSA, MD, Fellow, Department of Head and Neck Surgery, Roswell Park Cancer Institute, Buffalo, New York

GROESBECK P. PARHAM, MD, Professor (Obstetrics and Gynecology); and Avon Scholar for Cancer Control, Division of Gynecologic Oncology, University of Alabama at Birmingham, Birmingham, Alabama

NESTOR R. RIGUAL, MD, Associate Professor, Department of Head and Neck Surgery, Roswell Park Cancer Institute, Buffalo, New York

SHARON SPENCER, MD, Professor, Head and Neck Oncology, Department of Radiation, University of Alabama at Birmingham School of Medicine, Birmingham, Alabama

CHERYL L. WALKER, MD, President, The Kerr L. White Institute for Health Services Research, Duluth, Georgia

CARLTON J. YOUNG, MD, Associate Professor (Surgery); and Director, Pancreas Transplantation, Division of Transplantation, Department of Surgery, University of Alabama at Birmingham, Birmingham, Alabama

CONTENTS

Update on Disparities in the Pathophysiology and Management of Hypertension: Focus on African Americans   921

Crystal A. Gadegbeku, Janice P. Lea, and
Kenneth A. Jamerson

> Hypertension in African Americans accounts for excess cardiovascular morbidity and mortality. There is a disproportionate prevalence of hypertension in this population, and African Americans have benefited less than other populations from medical advancement. Over the decades, research has attempted to identify pathophysiology unique to this racial group. Emerging from clinical investigation focused on this patient population is the awareness that a complexity of factors interacts and converges, resulting in the increased disease expression and clinical sequelae. This review focuses on recent observations and insights, from genetic to environmental factors, associated with hypertension in African Americans and highlights evidence-based approaches to treatment that have demonstrated cardiovascular benefits in recent clinical trials.

Racial Disparities Affecting the Reproductive Health of African-American Women   935

Groesbeck P. Parham and Michael L. Hicks

> Racial disparities affecting the reproductive health of African-American women range from a twofold excess risk of delivering a preterm baby to a fourfold excess risk of maternal death. They extend from being subjected to unnecessary primary caesarean deliveries to receiving substandard surgical procedures, chemotherapy, and radiation for reproductive tract malignancies. What is it that puts African-American women at risk for such outcomes, and how can they be permanently eliminated? As substrate for the serious debate and conversation that needs to take place around the subject matter, this article discusses some of the most critical areas

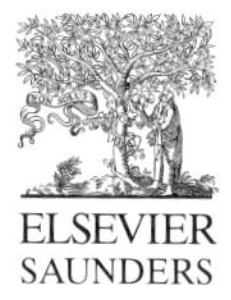

ELSEVIER
SAUNDERS

THE MEDICAL
CLINICS
OF NORTH AMERICA

Med Clin N Am 89 (2005) xi–xii

Preface

Minority Health and Disparities-Related Issues: Part II

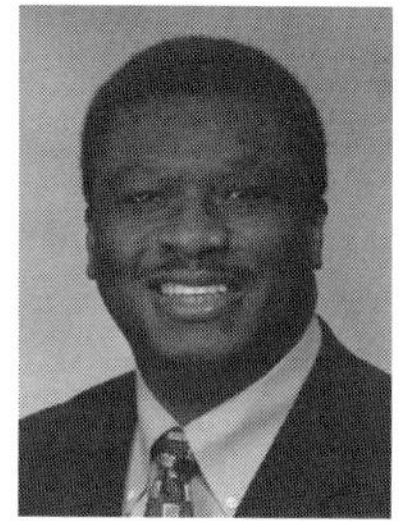

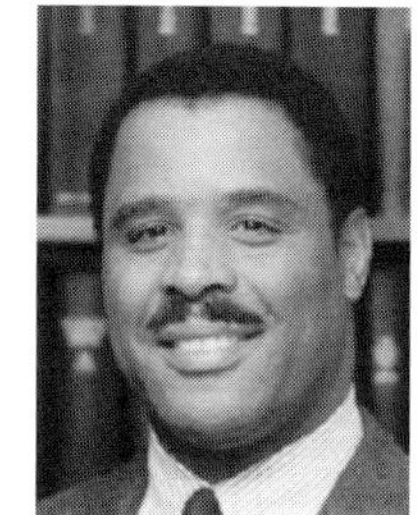

Eddie L. Greene, MD Charles R. Thomas, Jr., MD
Guest Editors

Our primary aim of this two-part issue of *Medical Clinics of North America* is to provide an evidence-based summary of the multifaceted problem of health care disparities that continue to present a challenge to health care providers and also appear to disproportionately affect identifiable segments of our society, mainly minority and underserved populations. Despite major technologic advances, ever more sophisticated pathophysiologic insights, and an increase in the numbers of health care providers, patients from minority populations and those with limited access to quality health care generally continue to have worse outcomes. For many of the major diseases affecting all Americans at the beginning of the 21st century, the rates of morbidity and mortality in minority populations continue to be excessive. These points are sobering, and moreover are poignantly illustrated in the data for heart disease, many types of cancer, diabetes, renal disease, pain management, and HIV/AIDS treatment. Questions persist about the reasons for health care disparities and are not easily answered. The epidemiologists have extensively provided the quantitative measures indicating how profound the problems are and moreover how they are projected to grow. We would like to suggest that now is the time to move beyond the statistics. Although extensive queries will continue to be important, practical answers may already lie in some of the existing genetic and pathophysiologic insights obtained from basic science and clinical investigations.

Recent advances in elucidating the human genome will help to redefine the limited biologic construct of race or ethnicity as a surrogate for genotype inter- and intra-population patient variation. Additional answers may be gained by evaluating new strategies for health care delivery and extensively evaluating the clinical and cognitive process that affect every day clinical decision-making when clinical investigators, practitioners and health care providers see patients from minority populations. The assembled contributors were charged with addressing the salient issues and providing a concise review of the pathophysiologic mechanisms, new treatment strategies, and new ways to educate our clinician colleagues as well as our patients. Our contributors are some the best and brightest investigators and practitioners in Medicine today. They have cogently contributed what we believe will prove to be outstanding insights. However this is only a beginning.

We hope that these issues inspire many more of our colleagues to seek additional insights and answers to the vexing issues of the health care disparity matrix. Our patients deserve the best we have to offer. A looming question is: What happens next?

We would like to thank all of our contributors for their outstanding efforts in making this a successful endeavor. We would also like to thank Heather Cullen, Rachel Glover, Alexandra Pastor, and others at Elsevier for their generous contributions of time, talent, expertise, and discipline to ensure an outstanding issue of *Medical Clinics of North America*.

Eddie L. Greene, MD
Division of Nephrology
Department of Internal Medicine
Mayo Clinic College of Medicine
200 First Street SW
Rochester, MN 55905, USA

E-mail address: Greene.eddie@mayo.edu

Charles R. Thomas, Jr., MD
Department of Radiation Oncology
San Antonio Cancer Institute
University of Texas Health Science Center at San Antonio
7979 Wurzbach Road
San Antonio, TX 78229, USA

E-mail address: cthomas@ctrc.net

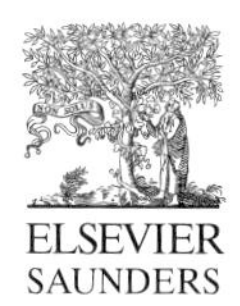

ELSEVIER
SAUNDERS

Med Clin N Am 89 (2005) 921–933

THE MEDICAL
CLINICS
OF NORTH AMERICA

Update on Disparities in the Pathophysiology and Management of Hypertension: Focus on African Americans

Crystal A. Gadegbeku, MD[a,*], Janice P. Lea, MD[b],
Kenneth A. Jamerson, MD[a]

[a]*Division of Nephrology, Department of Internal Medicine,
University of Michigan Health System, 310 Simpson Memorial Institute,
102 Observatory Road, Ann Arbor, MI, 48109-0725, USA*
[b]*Renal Division, Department of Medicine, Emory University School of Medicine,
1639 Pierce Drive, WMB Room 338, Atlanta, GA 30322, USA*

African Americans suffer earlier onset and higher prevalence and severity of hypertension than any other ethnic population in the United States [1]. These factors contribute to the excess cardiovascular morbidity and mortality observed in this racial group (Fig. 1) [2]. Compared with Americans of European descent, African Americans have a twofold higher incidence of stroke [3], a fourfold higher prevalence of hypertensive nephropathy [4], and a 50% higher mortality from heart disease [3]. Furthermore, cardiovascular disease morbidity and mortality have decreased less dramatically in African Americans [5]. An alarming recent observation is that despite the increasing prevalence and patient awareness of hypertension over the last 3 decades in all populations (but particularly in African Americans), blood pressure control rates are stagnant [6]. This phenomenon, along with the increasing rates of other comorbid conditions like obesity and diabetes, is likely to have cumulative effects on the already high burden of cardiovascular disease in African Americans.

A unifying pathophysiologic phenomenon that explains the rates of hypertension in African Americans has not been identified. Most likely, hypertension and its consequences are due to multiple factors (not necessarily linked to race per se) that converge in this patient population.

* Corresponding author.
E-mail address: cgadegbe@umich.edu (C.A. Gadegbeku).

0025-7125/05/$ - see front matter © 2005 Elsevier Inc. All rights reserved.
doi:10.1016/j.mcna.2005.05.003   *medical.theclinics.com*

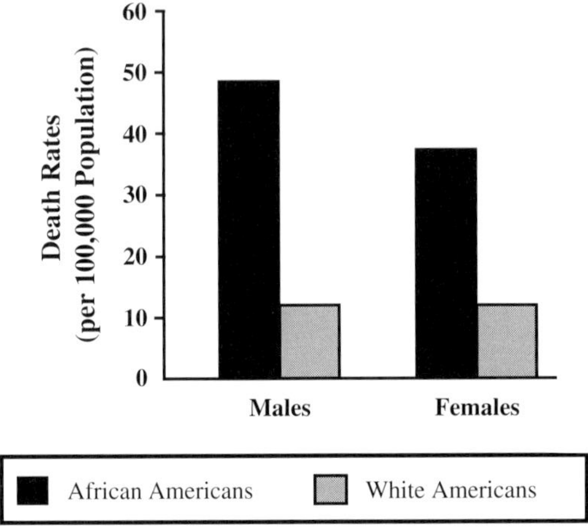

Fig. 1. Estimates of the number of deaths due to hypertension according to race. High blood pressure statistics, American Heart Association, 2004. (*Data from* Heart Disease and Stroke Statistical Update. Dallas (TX): American Heart Association; 2004. Available at: http://www. americanheart.org. © American Heart Association.)

Genetic epidemiology of hypertension in African Americans

Epidemiologic studies demonstrate that 20% to 70% of blood pressure characteristics are inherited [7,8]. The awareness of blood pressure heritablility has led to the concept that the disparate burden of hypertension in the African diaspora may principally be from a genetic predisposition. Consequently, there has been intensive formal investigation for candidate genes responsible for human hypertension, with several collaborative efforts focused on African Americans. The Middle Passage theory, a concept suggesting that a selection pressure driven by slavery resulted in survival of African Americans prone to hypertension [9], has not been supported in the literature. For example, sub-Saharan Africans have a prevalence of candidate genes similar to that of African Americans despite the significantly higher hypertension prevalence in the United States descendents [7,10]. Moreover, through genetic epidemiology research, it has been discovered that prevalence rates differ among the same ethnic groups from rural to westernized habitats, supporting the impact of the environment on potentially genetically susceptible populations [7]. Currently, experts in this field believe that hypertension is a polygenic disorder in which various clusters of gene mutations and multiple nongenetic factors are necessary for phenotypic expression.

Through intensive genetic research, multiple mutations have been identified; however, most of these mutations have unclear physiologic relevance most likely due to several limitations with previous approaches to identification of genetic defects in hypertension [7]. One issue is that gene abnormalities have been identified based on markers or "intermediate phenotypes" that are not clearly pathophysiologic. A second limitation is that most studies have focused on structural abnormalities, not on functional abnormalities. Third, although there is increasing awareness of the complexities of gene–gene and gene–environment interactions, there are not adequate analytic tools to carefully examine the influences of these factors. These limitations probably explain why gene polymorphisms described in the renin-angiotensin system, kallikrein-kinin system, and atrial natriuretic peptide are of little clinical significance [7]. In addition, mutations in the epithelial sodium channel (described later), hypothesized to be linked to salt-sensitive hypertension, have yielded conflicting results [11–13]. Therefore, identification of genes responsible for hypertension has proved difficult based on traditional methodologies. New technology using genome-wide scanning offers more promise and has identified several chromosomes linked with blood pressure and heart rate characteristics among African [14], African American, and white families [15,16] and kidney function in African Americans [17]. These observations have provided scientists with genetic "areas of interest" for future study. In this era of expanding investigation in pharmacogenomics, the identification of gene-specific defects has the potential to lead to effective targeted and individualized treatment for all patients. At this point, however, there is no clear evidence indicating that African Americans, as a racial group, have a unique hypertensive disorder on a genetic basis.

New insight into pathophysiology

The renin-angiotensin system paradox

Low renin levels are a well-established characteristic of hypertension in this population. The suppression of renin has been considered a secondary response to sodium retention and volume excess. Along these lines, it was thought that the renin-angiotensin system was not a key contributor of hypertension in African Americans. Recent renal hemodynamic studies in African Americans revealed that compared with white subjects, renal plasma flow is reduced with blunted pressor responses to angiotensin II along with enhanced vasodilator responses to angiotensin II–converting enzyme inhibitors. Collectively, these observations suggest that there may be enhanced intrarenal activation of the renin-angiotensin system [18]. Potentially, increased tissue levels of angiotensin II, which cannot be measured in humans, lead to feedback inhibition of plasma renin levels. The enhanced local renin-angiotensin system activity could contribute to hypertension and target-organ injury, particularly in the kidney. Further, increased activity of the intrarenal renin-angiotensin system may explain the enhanced susceptibility of African Americans to all forms of nephropathy. As described later, the renin-angiotensin system paradox is supported by the long-term beneficial effects of the renin-angiotensin system blockade in clinical trials and should lead to further therapeutic trials in this population.

Salt sensitivity in African Americans

Salt sensitivity, defined as an increase in blood pressure in response to a high-salt diet, is more commonly described in normotensive and hypertensive African Americans [19,20]. Recently, clinical research in populations of African descent has focused on potential defects in renal sodium transport to explain this hemodynamic phenomenon. More interest in this area has been generated by the identification of mutations in the amiloride-sensitive epithelial sodium channel in the rare hypertensive disorder, Liddle syndrome. As in Liddle syndrome, hypertensive patients who have T594M, an epithelial sodium channel mutation, have been successfully treated with amiloride, a diuretic that specifically blocks epithelial sodium channel sodium reabsorption [11]. Black South Africans who have the T594M polymorphism, however, do not have an increased prevalence of hypertension [12]. Alternately, Afro-Caribbeans who have essential hypertension did not show abnormalities in the epithelial sodium channel gene [13]. In addition, amiloride did not lower blood pressure in blacks as effectively as in whites [21]. Theoretically, enhanced epithelial sodium channel activity should lead to enhanced potassium excretion, and African Americans have reduced urinary potassium levels at various levels of potassium intake [18,22]. Epithelial sodium channel mutations, therefore, have not explained the high prevalence of salt sensitivity in African Americans; however, dysregulation of other renal sodium transport mechanisms are being investigated [22]. There is also evidence that other hormonal abnormalities related to salt sensitivity, like diminished kallikrein–kinin biosynthesis [22] and reduced nitric oxide [23,24], have been described in African Americans.

A salient factor contributing to salt-sensitive hypertension in all populations studied is obesity [25]. Epidemiologic evidence demonstrates an increasing prevalence of obesity in America and worldwide. As in other populations, obesity has significantly impacted on the prevalence of hypertension in people of the African diaspora (Fig. 2) [26]. Recent epidemiologic data estimate that 70% and 77% of African-American men and women, respectively, are overweight [27]. These observations are consistent with the increased prevalence of hypertension and suggest that culture and environment are equally if not more important than other factors. This high prevalence of obesity highlights the importance of lifestyle-modification strategies that are challenging and often-ignored aspects of the treatment plan.

Vascular function in African Americans

Hypertension in all populations, including African Americans [28], is typically characterized by high systemic vascular resistance. The high

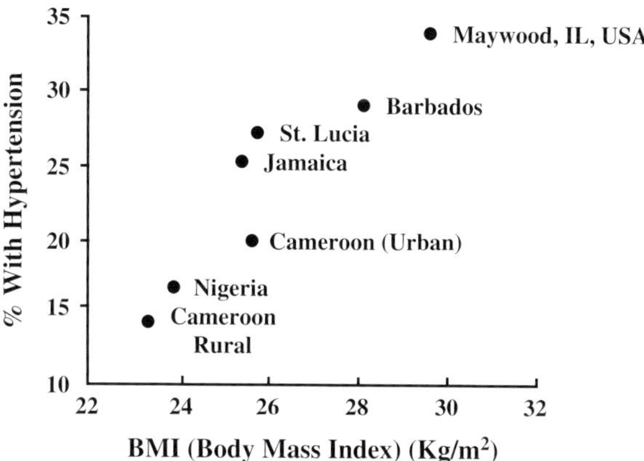

Fig. 2. Relationship of body mass index to hypertension prevalence in populations of West African origin. (*Adapted from* Cooper R, Rotimi C. Hypertension in blacks. Am J Hypertens 1997;10:213; with permission.)

burden of vascular disease has led to research examining vasomotor function in African Americans. It has been suggested that sympathetic overactivity is a feature of hypertension in African Americans [9]. In support of previous data, recent research demonstrates that vasoconstrictor responses to various adrenergic stimuli are enhanced in this hypertensive population [29–31]. Moreover, African Americans may be susceptible to impairment of the endothelium, which has a major role in vascular homeostasis. Endothelin is a potent vasoconstrictor hormone produced by the endothelium that acts on vascular smooth muscle. Higher levels of endothelin are found in African Americans who have hypertension [32]; these levels are increased during mental stress [33] and correlate with increases in vascular tone in normo- and hypertensive individuals [34].

From another perspective, enhanced vasoconstriction may, in part, be a manifestation of impaired vasodilation. Several groups have demonstrated abnormalities in endothelium-dependent vasodilation in normotensive and hypertensive blacks using several different techniques [29,35–40]. Further, Houghton and colleagues [41] noted reduced nitric oxide–mediated vasodilation and enhanced coronary blood flow responses to the nitric oxide precursor L-arginine in coronaries of hypertensive blacks with left ventricular hypertrophy. This finding suggests that selective groups of African Americans may be prone to reduced vascular nitric oxide bio-availability. Nitric oxide deficiency leads to multiple events implicated in vascular disease and may therefore be an important abnormality contributing to the high cardiovascular disease burden in African Americans. In addition, reduced plasma nitric oxide levels [23,24] and increased levels of its inhibitor, asymmetric dimethlyarginine [24], are associated with salt sensitivity. In support of the theory of reduced nitric oxide bioavailability, there is clinical evidence that African Americans who have congestive heart failure receive significant benefit from nitrovasodilator therapy [42]. Some studies have also noted impairment in endothelium-independent vasodilation [40,43]. These findings suggest that vascular abnormalities extend beyond the endothelium and raise the possibility that observations of abnormal vascular function may be manifestations of subclinical vascular disease and hence, a pathophysiologic consequence and not a cause of abnormal blood pressure regulation.

Psychosocial issues in hypertension in African Americans

Social issues clearly contribute to the high prevalence of hypertension in African Americans. One of 4 African Americans is below the poverty level compared with 1 of 12 white Americans. Clearly, low socioeconomic status is identified as a risk factor for hypertension in many populations. Low socioeconomic status is linked to increased stress, poor nutrition, obesity, and increased tobacco and alcohol use, which may have cumulative effects leading to hypertension. In addition, nutritional factors such as low intake of fresh fruits, vegetables, and milk (rich in potassium and calcium) substantially influence blood pressure. Therefore, the direct impact of daily economic and social stress and the consequences of coping behavioral strategies are important factors in the development of hypertension and its high prevalence rates in African Americans. Lifestyle modifications, recently summarized (Table 1) [44] and successfully implemented in community-based programs [45], have proved to have short- and long-term benefit in the treatment of hypertension. In addition, transcendental meditation and relaxation techniques in controlled trials produced reduction in systolic and

Table 1
Lifestyle modification to manage hypertension

Modification	Recommendation	Reduction in systolic blood pressure
Weight reduction	Maintain BMI between 18.5–24.9 kg/m^2	5–20 mm Hg/10 kg of weight loss
Adopt DASH diet	Consume diet rich in fruits and vegetables and low in saturated fats	8–14 mm Hg
Dietary sodium reduction	Reduce sodium intake to $\leq$ 100 mEq/L	2–8 mm Hg
Phyical activity	At least 30 min of exercise most days of the week	4–9 mm Hg
Moderation of ethanol consumption	Limit consumprtion to 2 drinks in men and 1 drink in women	2–4 mm Hg

Abbreviations: BMI, body mass index; DASH, dietary approach to stop hypertension.
Data from Chobanian AV, Bakris GL, Black HR, et al. Seventh report of the Joint National Committee on Prevention, Detection, Evaluation, and Treatment of High Blood Pressure. Hypertension 2003;42:1206–52.

diastolic blood pressure of 5 to 10 mm Hg and 3 to 6 mm Hg, respectively, in African Americans in the range of pharmacologic interventions [46,47]. For successful treatment of hypertension in African Americans, significant attention should be directed toward strategies to manage or reduce the impact of these issues.

Approach to pharmacologic therapy

Given the greater prevalence of hypertension and risk of cardiovascular complications in the African-American population, a compelling argument could be made to setting more aggressive blood pressure goals for African Americans. None of the large-scale clinical trials [48] to date, however, has demonstrated a significant cardiovascular benefit by achieving blood pressure targets below 120/80 mm Hg in most hypertensive subjects, even those at high risk for cardiovascular disease. The African-American Study of Kidney Disease and Hypertension trial [49] prospectively sought to determine the impact of achieving a blood pressure target below 120/80 mm Hg in patients who have hypertensive nephropathy. African Americans achieved renal and cardiovascular outcomes similar to those in the usual-goal treatment group (blood pressure < 140/90 mm Hg). These results suggest that the current guidelines for the general population stipulated by the seventh report of the Joint National Committee on Detection, Prevention, Evaluation, and Treatment of High Blood Pressure (JNC 7) are applicable to African Americans (Fig 3A) [50]. The Hypertension in African Americans Working Group has issued a consensus statement that includes management guidelines comparable to the JNC 7 recommendations (Fig. 3B) [51]. Specifically, lifestyle intervention, as outlined in both management algorithms (see Fig. 3) and in detail in Table 1, should be formally implemented in subjects when blood pressure is greater than 120/80 mm Hg and pharmacologic therapy should be added when blood pressure exceeds 140/90 mm Hg. A combination of two drugs is indicated when blood pressure is 160/100 mm Hg or greater. As evidenced by large clinical trials, most patients of all ethnic backgrounds required two to four agents to achieve systolic and diastolic blood pressure goals defined by the JNC 7 [48,52–55].

With regard to monotherapy, a meta-analysis of randomized controlled trials of various agents in hypertensive patients of African descent demonstrates reductions of 3 to 15 mm Hg in systolic blood pressure and 2 to 10 mm Hg in diastolic blood pressure [56]. In this analysis, calcium channel blockers appeared to have the greatest effect at all stages of hypertension, including in patients who have diastolic blood pressures greater than 110 mm Hg. Among the other classes of antihypertensive agents, diuretics, central sympatholytics, α-blockers, and angiotensin II receptor blockers appeared to be more effective than β-blockers and angiotensin-converting enzyme inhibitors at lowering blood pressure [56]. Another

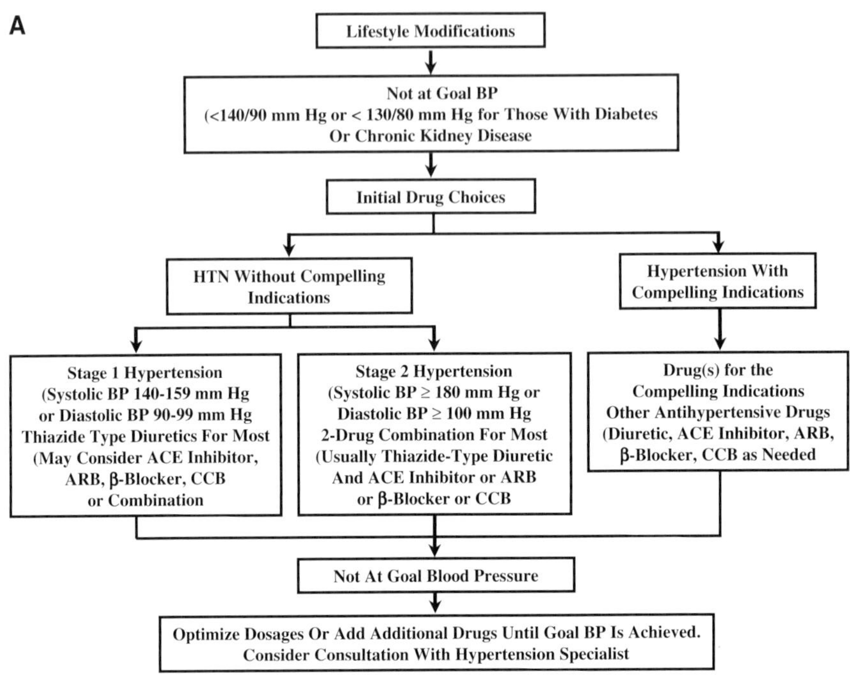
A
Lifestyle Modifications
Not at Goal BP
(<140/90 mm Hg or < 130/80 mm Hg for Those With Diabetes
Or Chronic Kidney Disease
Initial Drug Choices
HTN Without Compelling
Indications
Hypertension With
Compelling Indications
Stage 1 Hypertension
(Systolic BP 140-159 mm Hg
or Diastolic BP 90-99 mm Hg
Thiazide Type Diuretics For Most
(May Consider ACE Inhibitor,
ARB, β-Blocker, CCB
or Combination
Stage 2 Hypertension
(Systolic BP ≥ 180 mm Hg or
Diastolic BP ≥ 100 mm Hg
2-Drug Combination For Most
(Usually Thiazide-Type Diuretic
And ACE Inhibitor or ARB
or β-Blocker or CCB
Drug(s) for the
Compelling Indications
Other Antihypertensive Drugs
(Diuretic, ACE Inhibitor, ARB,
β-Blocker, CCB as Needed
Not At Goal Blood Pressure
Optimize Dosages Or Add Additional Drugs Until Goal BP Is Achieved.
Consider Consultation With Hypertension Specialist

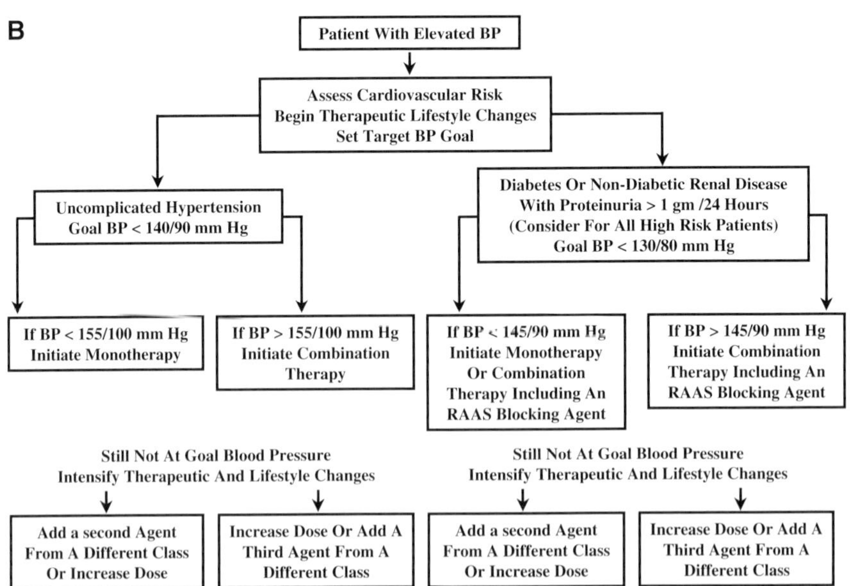
B
Patient With Elevated BP
Assess Cardiovascular Risk
Begin Therapeutic Lifestyle Changes
Set Target BP Goal
Uncomplicated Hypertension
Goal BP < 140/90 mm Hg
Diabetes Or Non-Diabetic Renal Disease
With Proteinuria > 1 gm /24 Hours
(Consider For All High Risk Patients)
Goal BP < 130/80 mm Hg
If BP < 155/100 mm Hg
Initiate Monotherapy
If BP > 155/100 mm Hg
Initiate Combination
Therapy
If BP < 145/90 mm Hg
Initiate Monotherapy
Or Combination
Therapy Including An
RAAS Blocking Agent
If BP > 145/90 mm Hg
Initiate Combination
Therapy Including An
RAAS Blocking Agent
Still Not At Goal Blood Pressure
Intensify Therapeutic And Lifestyle Changes
Still Not At Goal Blood Pressure
Intensify Therapeutic And Lifestyle Changes
Add a second Agent
From A Different Class
Or Increase Dose
Increase Dose Or Add A
Third Agent From A
Different Class
Add a second Agent
From A Different Class
Or Increase Dose
Increase Dose Or Add A
Third Agent From A
Different Class
Not At Goal With Three Agents.
Consider Factors That May Decrease Compliance Or Efficacy With The Current Regimen
Consider Consultation With Hypertension Specialist

meta-analysis of 15 clinical trials comparing black–white variations in drug efficacy determined that blood pressure responses and variations in responses to all drug classes were similar in these ethnic groups [57]. In some studies, African Americans had higher baseline blood pressures, resulting in significantly lower "success" rates of treatment-to-goal outcomes; however, actual blood pressure reductions were equivalent to those of whites. Furthermore, when agents are combined, which is necessary for most patients, there are even fewer, if any, racial differences [58,59]. Notably, low-dose combination therapy, recommended for blood pressure 160/100 mm Hg or greater, is associated with fewer side effects than dose-titration of monotherapy [44]. Given the need for more than one antihypertensive agent, fixed-dose combination products (combining diuretics with angiotensin-converting enzyme inhibitors, angiotensin II receptor blockers, or β-blockers and combining calcium channel blockers with angiotensin-converting enzyme inhibitors) are commercially available and reduce concerns about compliance.

Reduction in blood pressure is an important clinical measure, however, the ultimate goal is optimal target-organ protection. Although the pathobiology of hypertension suggests that specific mechanisms for lowering blood pressure (ie, blocking the renin-angiotensin system) ought to yield superior outcomes, to date, a preponderance of the clinical trial data suggests that it is lowering blood pressure and not the specific agent used that imparts most of the cardiovascular protection to hypertensive subjects. The Antihypertensive and Lipid-Lowering Treatment to Prevent Heart Attacks (ALLHAT) trial demonstrated that chlorthalidone, a thiazide-type diuretic, was very effective at reducing cardiovascular events and controlling blood pressure in black participants (35% of the study population) [60,61]. The diuretic therapy was also the most effective agent in lowering blood pressure in African Americans. On the other hand, initial therapy with an α-blocker was associated with poorer blood pressure control, increased side effects, and lack of cardiovascular benefit.

Fig. 3. (*A*) Clinical algorithm recommended by the Joint National Committee on the treatment of hypertension (JNC 7 report). (*Adapted from* Chobanian AV, Bakris GL, Black HR, et al. The seventh report of the Joint National Committee on Prevention, Detection, Evaluation, and Treatment of High Blood Pressure: the JNC 7 report. JAMA 2003;289:2564; with permission.) (*B*) Clinical algorithm for achieving target blood pressure in African Americans recommended by the Hypertension in African Americans Working Group. Note the similarities in consensus guidelines for the general population and African-American population. (*From* Douglas JG, Bakris GL, Epstein M, et al. Management of high blood pressure in African Americans: consensus statement of the Hypertension in African Americans Working Group of the International Society on Hypertension in Blacks. Arch Intern Med 2003;163:532; with permission.) ACE, angiotensin-converting enzyme; ARB, angiotensin II receptor blocker; BP, blood pressure; CCB, calcium channel blocker; HTN, hypertension; RAAS, renin-angiotensin-aldosterone system.

Recent clinical trials, which have included more diverse populations than in the past, support that African Americans derive a benefit similar to majority patients from agents prescribed for specific indications. For instance, the African-American Study of Kidney Disease and Hypertension trial, designed to examine antihypertensive treatment solely in African Americans who have hypertensive nephropathy, confirmed that angiotensin-converting enzyme inhibitors are superior to β-blockers and amlodipine in preventing renal progression [49]. In addition, trials that had 25% to 30% enrollment of African Americans have confirmed that β-blockers are beneficial in patients who have heart failure [62] and after myocardial infarction [63]. Therefore, the clinical outcomes of treatment aimed at reducing cardiovascular disease appear to be no different in African Americans than in other populations. These observations stress the importance of initial and ongoing clinical assessment of risk and target-organ involvement in developing the appropriate therapeutic strategy in this high-risk population.

Summary

Hypertension treatment and control is of paramount importance in the prevention of premature cardiovascular disease. African Americans present a special challenge to the clinician due, in part, to their earlier age of onset, greater prevalence, and increased rates of untoward events.

A review of the recent studies of genetic epidemiology has not revealed unique genotypes that explain human hypertension or the disparate impact suffered by African Americans. Moreover, a clear message has emerged that environmental factors predominate in their effect on cardiovascular risk and are mutable. These findings suggest that to have an immediate and substantial impact on the ethnic disparity of hypertension, resources and research should be directed toward social and behavioral factors. Prompt and aggressive control of blood pressure is an effective global strategy for cardiovascular risk reduction. In most cases, this approach requires multiple interventions including lifestyle modification and an antihypertensive regimen that is tailored to the individual under the current guidelines and not stipulated by race.

References

[1] Cooper RS, Liao Y, Rotimi C. Is hypertension more severe among US blacks, or is severe hypertension more common? Ann Epidemiol 1996;6:173–80.
[2] Kuller LH. Cardiovascular diseases and stroke in African-Americans and other racial minorities in the United States. A statement for health professionals. Introduction. Circulation 1991;83:1463–5.

[3] Heart Disease and Stroke Statistical Update. Dallas (TX): American Heart Association; 2004. Available at: http://www.americanheart.org.

[4] USRDS: the United States Renal Data System. Am J Kidney Dis 2003;42:1–230.

[5] Martins D, Norris K. Hypertension treatment in African Americans: physiology is less important than sociology. Cleve Clin J Med 2004;71:735–43.

[6] Glover M, Greenlund KJ, Ayala C, et al. Racial/ethnic disparities in prevalence, treatment, and control of hypertension—United States, 1999–2002. Centers for Disease Control and Prevention. MMWR Morb Mortal Wkly Rep 2005;54:57–9.

[7] Daniel HI, Rotimi CN. Genetic epidemiology of hypertension: an update on the African diaspora. Ethn Dis 2003;13:S53–66.

[8] Lifton RP, Gharavi AG, Geller DS. Molecular mechanisms of human hypertension. Cell 2001;104:545–56.

[9] Fray JCS, Douglas JG. Pathophysiology of hypertension in blacks. New York: Oxford University Press; 1993.

[10] Poston WS, Pavlik VN, Hyman DJ, et al. Genetic bottlenecks, perceived racism, and hypertension risk among African Americans and first-generation African immigrants. J Hum Hypertens 2001;15:341–51.

[11] Swift PA, Macgregor GA. Genetic variation in the epithelial sodium channel: a risk factor for hypertension in people of African origin. Adv Ren Replace Ther 2004;11: 76–86.

[12] Nkeh B, Samani NJ, Badenhorst D, et al. T594M variant of the epithelial sodium channel beta-subunit gene and hypertension in individuals of African ancestry in South Africa. Am J Hypertens 2003;16:847–52.

[13] Munroe PB, Strautnieks SS, Farrall M, et al. Absence of linkage of the epithelial sodium channel to hypertension in black Caribbeans. Am J Hypertens 1998;11:942–5.

[14] Cooper RS, Luke A, Zhu X, et al. Genome scan among Nigerians linking blood pressure to chromosomes 2, 3, and 19. Hypertension 2002;40:629–33.

[15] Rice T, Rankinen T, Chagnon YC, et al. Genomewide linkage scan of resting blood pressure: HERITAGE Family Study. Health, risk factors, exercise training, and genetics. Hypertension 2002;39:1037–43.

[16] Wilk JB, Myers RH, Zhang Y, et al. Evidence for a gene influencing heart rate on chromosome 4 among hypertensives. Hum Genet 2002;111:207–13.

[17] DeWan AT, Arnett DK, Atwood LD, et al. A genome scan for renal function among hypertensives: the HyperGEN study. Am J Hum Genet 2001;68:136–44.

[18] Price DA, Fisher ND. The renin-angiotensin system in blacks: active, passive, or what? Curr Hypertens Rep 2003;5:225–30.

[19] Sowers JR, Zemel MB, Zemel P, et al. Salt sensitivity in blacks. Salt intake and natriuretic substances. Hypertension 1988;12:485–90.

[20] Brier ME, Luft FC. Sodium kinetics in white and black normotensive subjects: possible relevance to salt-sensitive hypertension. Am J Med Sci 1994;307(Suppl 1):S38–42.

[21] Pratt JH, Ambrosius WT, Agarwal R, et al. Racial difference in the activity of the amiloride-sensitive epithelial sodium channel. Hypertension 2002;40:903–8.

[22] Aviv A, Hollenberg NK, Weder A. Urinary potassium excretion and sodium sensitivity in blacks. Hypertension 2004;43:707–13.

[23] Campese VM, Mozayeni P, Ye S, et al. High salt intake inhibits nitric oxide synthase expression and aggravates hypertension in rats with chronic renal failure. J Nephrol 2002;15: 407–13.

[24] Fujiwara N, Osanai T, Kamada T, et al. Study on the relationship between plasma nitrite and nitrate level and salt sensitivity in human hypertension: modulation of nitric oxide synthesis by salt intake. Circulation 2000;101:856–61.

[25] Rocchini AP. Obesity hypertension, salt sensitivity and insulin resistance. Nutr Metab Cardiovasc Dis 2000;10:287–94.

[26] Cooper R, Rotimi C. Hypertension in blacks. Am J Hypertens 1997;10:804–12.

[27] Flegal KM, Carroll MD, Ogden CL, et al. Prevalence and trends in obesity among US adults, 1999–2000. JAMA 2002;288:1723–7.

[28] Rockstroh JK, Schmieder RE, Schlaich MP, et al. Renal and systemic hemodynamics in black and white hypertensive patients. Am J Hypertens 1997;10:971–8.

[29] Stein CM, Lang CC, Nelson R, et al. Vasodilation in black Americans: attenuated nitric oxide-mediated responses. Clin Pharmacol Ther 1997;62:436–43.

[30] Sherwood A, Hinderliter AL. Responsiveness to alpha- and beta-adrenergic receptor agonists. Effects of race in borderline hypertensive compared to normotensive men. Am J Hypertens 1993;6:630–5.

[31] Eichler HG, Blaschke TF, Hoffman BB. Decreased responsiveness of superficial hand veins to phenylephrine in black normotensive males. J Cardiovasc Pharmacol 1990;16: 177–81.

[32] Ergul A. Hypertension in black patients: an emerging role of the endothelin system in salt-sensitive hypertension. Hypertension 2000;36:62–7.

[33] Treiber FA, Jackson RW, Davis H, et al. Racial differences in endothelin-1 at rest and in response to acute stress in adolescent males. Hypertension 2000;35:722–5.

[34] Campia U, Cardillo C, Panza JA. Ethnic differences in the vasoconstrictor activity of endogenous endothelin-1 in hypertensive patients. Circulation 2004;109:3191–5.

[35] Perregaux D, Chaudhuri A, Rao S, et al. Brachial vascular reactivity in blacks. Hypertension 2000;36:866–71.

[36] Jones DS, Andrawis NS, Abernethy DR. Impaired endothelial-dependent forearm vascular relaxation in black Americans. Clin Pharmacol Ther 1999;65:408–12.

[37] Houghton JL, Smith VE, Strogatz DS, et al. Effect of African-American race and hypertensive left ventricular hypertrophy on coronary vascular reactivity and endothelial function. Hypertension 1997;29:706–14.

[38] Kahn DF, Duffy SJ, Tomasian D, et al. Effects of black race on forearm resistance vessel function. Hypertension 2002;40:195–201.

[39] Vita JA. Nitric oxide and vascular reactivity in African American patients with hypertension. J Card Fail 2003;9:S199–204 [discussion: S205].

[40] Campia U, Choucair WK, Bryant MB, et al. Reduced endothelium-dependent and -independent dilation of conductance arteries in African Americans. J Am Coll Cardiol 2002; 40:754–60.

[41] Houghton JL, Philbin EF, Strogatz DS, et al. The presence of African American race predicts improvement in coronary endothelial function after supplementary L-arginine. J Am Coll Cardiol 2002;39:1314–22.

[42] Taylor AL, Ziesche S, Yancy C, et al. Combination of isosorbide dinitrate and hydralazine in blacks with heart failure. N Engl J Med 2004;351:2049–57.

[43] Stein CM, Lang CC, Singh I, et al. Increased vascular adrenergic vasoconstriction and decreased vasodilation in blacks. Additive mechanisms leading to enhanced vascular reactivity. Hypertension 2000;36:945–51.

[44] Chobanian AV, Bakris GL, Black HR, et al. Seventh report of the Joint National Committee on Prevention, Detection, Evaluation, and Treatment of High Blood Pressure. Hypertension 2003;42:1206–52.

[45] Oexmann MJ, Ascanio R, Egan BM. Efficacy of a church-based intervention on cardiovascular risk reduction. Ethn Dis 2001;11:817–22.

[46] Barnes V, Schneider R, Alexander C, et al. Stress, stress reduction, and hypertension in African Americans: an updated review. J Natl Med Assoc 1997;89:464–76.

[47] Schneider RH, Staggers F, Alxander CN, et al. A randomised controlled trial of stress reduction for hypertension in older African Americans. Hypertension 1995;26:820–7.

[48] Hansson L, Zanchetti A, Carruthers SG, et al. Effects of intensive blood-pressure lowering and low-dose aspirin in patients with hypertension: principal results of the Hypertension Optimal Treatment (HOT) randomised trial. HOT Study Group. Lancet 1998;351:1755–62.

[49] Agodoa LY, Appel L, Bakris GL, et al. Effect of ramipril vs amlodipine on renal outcomes in hypertensive nephrosclerosis: a randomized controlled trial. JAMA 2001;285:2719–28.

[50] Chobanian AV, Bakris GL, Black HR, et al. The seventh report of the Joint National Committee on Prevention, Detection, Evaluation, and Treatment of High Blood Pressure: the JNC 7 report. JAMA 2003;289:2560–72.

[51] Douglas JG, Bakris GL, Epstein M, et al. Management of high blood pressure in African Americans: consensus statement of the Hypertension in African Americans Working Group of the International Society on Hypertension in Blacks. Arch Intern Med 2003;163:525–41.

[52] Major outcomes in high-risk hypertensive patients randomized to angiotensin-converting enzyme inhibitor or calcium channel blocker vs diuretic: the Antihypertensive and Lipid-Lowering Treatment to Prevent Heart Attack Trial (ALLHAT). JAMA 2002;288:2981–97.

[53] Hansson L, Lindholm LH, Ekbom T, et al. Randomised trial of old and new anti-hypertensive drugs in elderly patients: cardiovascular mortality and morbidity the Swedish Trial in Old Patients with Hypertension-2 study. Lancet 1999;354:1751–6.

[54] Prevention of stroke by antihypertensive drug treatment in older persons with isolated systolic hypertension. Final results of the Systolic Hypertension in the Elderly Program (SHEP). SHEP Cooperative Research Group. JAMA 1991;265:3255–64.

[55] Staessen JA, Fagard R, Thijs L, et al. Randomised double-blind comparison of placebo and active treatment for older patients with isolated systolic hypertension. The Systolic Hypertension in Europe (Syst-Eur) Trial Investigators. Lancet 1997;350:757–64.

[56] Brewster LM, van Montfrans GA, Kleijnen J. Systematic review: antihypertensive drug therapy in black patients. Ann Intern Med 2004;141:614–27.

[57] Sehgal AR. Overlap between whites and blacks in response to antihypertensive drugs. Hypertension 2004;43:566–72.

[58] Prisant LM, Mensah GA. Use of beta-adrenergic receptor blockers in blacks. J Clin Pharmacol 1996;36:867–73.

[59] Racial differences in response to low-dose captopril are abolished by the addition of hydrochlorothiazide. Br J Clin Pharmacol 1982;14(Suppl 2):97S–101S.

[60] Major cardiovascular events in hypertensive patients randomized to doxazosin vs chlorthalidone: the antihypertensive and lipid-lowering treatment to prevent heart attack trial (ALLHAT). ALLHAT Collaborative Research Group. JAMA 2000;283:1967–75.

[61] Lopes AA, James SA, Port FK, et al. Meeting the challenge to improve the treatment of hypertension in blacks. J Clin Hypertens (Greenwich) 2003;5:393–401.

[62] Yancy CW, Fowler MB, Colucci WS, et al. Race and the response to adrenergic blockade with carvedilol in patients with chronic heart failure. N Engl J Med 2001;344:1358–65.

[63] Gottlieb SS, McCarter RJ, Vogel RA. Effect of beta-blockade on mortality among high-risk and low-risk patients after myocardial infarction. N Engl J Med 1998;339:489–97.

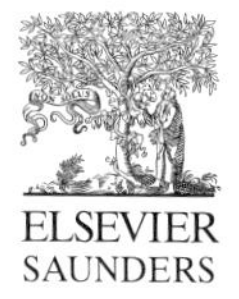

ELSEVIER
SAUNDERS

THE MEDICAL
CLINICS
OF NORTH AMERICA

Med Clin N Am 89 (2005) 935–943

Racial Disparities Affecting the Reproductive Health of African-American Women

Groesbeck P. Parham, MD[a],*, Michael L. Hicks, MD[b]

[a]*Division of Gynecologic Oncology, University of Alabama at Birmingham, OHB 538, 619 19th Street South, Birmingham, AL 35249–7333, USA*
[b]*Gynecologic Oncology, Michigan Cancer Institute, 44405 Woodward Avenue, Pontiac, MI 48341, USA*

Racial disparities affecting the reproductive health of African-American women range from a twofold excess risk of delivering a preterm baby to a fourfold excess risk of maternal death. They extend from being subjected to unnecessary primary caesarean deliveries [1] to receiving substandard surgical procedures, chemotherapy, and radiation for reproductive tract malignancies. The question that must ultimately be answered is this: "What is it that puts African-American women at risk for such outcomes, and how can they be permanently eliminated"? It is equally important that the ability to distinguish disparities from differences be developed. Just as important is the ability to know what problems can be solved by changing the environment (ie, access, education, transportation, and so forth) versus those that require some aspect of personal responsibility or lifestyle changes on the part of the potential client. As substrate for the serious debate and conversation that needs to take place around the subject matter, some of the most critical areas affecting the reproductive health of African-American women have been selected and the crucial aspects of the racial-related disparities are presented.

Infertility

According to National Survey of Family Growth data, approximately 60 million women in the United States are of reproductive age (15–44

---

* Corresponding author.
E-mail address: gparham@uabmc.edu (G.P. Parham).

doi:10.1016/j.mcna.2005.04.001 *medical.theclinics.com*

years) [2]. Of these women 15% reported use of some kind of fertility service in their lifetime, including medical advice, tests, drugs, surgery, or other treatments. Excluding women who were surgical sterile, rates of infertility were 6.4% for white women and 10.5% for African-American women. According to a recent survey, women most likely to seek fertility services were characterized as follows: non-Hispanic white, married, income 300% above poverty level, private health insurance holders in the last year, and college graduates [3]. Of the few studies that have examined the influence of race on the success of infertility treatment, one of the most informative is the investigation by Sharara and McClamrock [4], which evaluated differences in in vitro fertilization outcomes between white and African-American women in an inner-city program. In this study, African Americans made up over one fourth of the patients and they were found to have the following distinguishing characteristics in relationship to their white counterparts: (1) the duration of their infertility was longer, (2) they had a higher incidence of fallopian tube disease, (3) their body mass index was greater, (4) they required more aggressive ovarian stimulation, (5) their implantation rates were lower, and (6) they were three times less likely to become pregnant. More recently, an analysis of data compiled by the Society for Assisted Reproductive Technology (1999, 2000) [5] revealed a 21% lower live birth rate after in vitro fertilization for African-American women compared with white or Hispanic women of any race, when controlled for age. Additionally, African-American women had more infertility diagnoses than white women and were more likely to have a miscarriage after they became pregnant. These differences only appeared when comparing fresh and not frozen embryos.

There are many factors that determine whether a person seeks elective health care services but infertility carries its own unique manifestations and may impact disparities related to access. For instance, there are data that seem to indicate that African-American women, in general, may be more reluctant [2,3,6] to seek infertility services, such as assisted reproductive technology, because of the following cultural beliefs: (1) religious beliefs that such technologies are counter to God's wishes [7,8]; (2) distrust of the medical system stemming from involuntary sterilization and past and present mistreatment of African Americans; and (3) the extended family ethos in the African-American community, which embraces informal (or formal) adoption of the children of close relatives (eg, nieces, nephews) for whom their biologic parents may not be able to offer care, as opposed to artificially induced births [7,8].

It is estimated that approximately 22% of the unmet needs for infertility services are concentrated among the poor [3]. Because of their disproportionate representation among the poor, African Americans of low socioeconomic status are hampered in their ability to access assisted reproductive technology, which tends to be extremely expensive.

Maternal mortality

Maternal mortality rate is the number of maternal deaths per 100,000 live-born infants. In the United States the risk for maternal death has consistently been higher among African-American women than white women [9,10]. In a recent report by the Centers for Disease Control and Prevention, maternal mortality rates were calculated for 1987 to 1996 using information from birth and death certificates filed in state vital statistics offices and compiled by the Centers for Disease Control and Prevention's National Center for Health Statistics [11,12]. Maternal deaths were defined as deaths that occurred during pregnancy or within 42 days after pregnancy termination, regardless of pregnancy duration and site, from any cause related to or aggravated by the pregnancy, but not from accidental or incidental causes. During the period under consideration, the maternal mortality rate was higher for African-American women than white women in every state where ratios could be reliably calculated. More specifically, the maternal mortality rate for African-American women was three to six times higher than for white women and the African American/white ratio ranged from 2.6 to 6.3. To discern possible trends in maternal mortality, data were divided into two 5-year periods (1987–1991 and 1992–1996). For each time period the maternal mortality rate did not differ significantly for African-American women (18.8 and 20.3, respectively) or for white women (5.5 and 5, respectively). The proposed 2010 objective for maternal mortality using vital statistics data remains at 3.3 per 100,000 live-born infants. Although no overall national progress has been made in achieving this objective, for white women the goal has been achieved in three states (Massachusetts, Nebraska, and Washington) and has almost been met in eight other states (maternal mortality rates < 4). This is concrete evidence that, in the United States, lower levels of maternal mortality can be achieved.

Although African-American women have the highest risk for dying from every pregnancy-related cause of death reported and prenatal care reduces these risks, health-care access and use do not explain fully the disproportionate risk for maternal death for African-American women [13]. Other factors, such as the quality of care and interaction between health-seeking behaviors and satisfaction with care, may also explain part of this disparity.

Preterm births

National infant mortality rates among non-Hispanic African-American women are twice those of non-Hispanic white women [14]. Nearly two thirds of this disparity is attributable to a higher rate of preterm delivery (PTD) (ie, ≤ 37 weeks' gestation) among African Americans [15]. The Centers for Disease Control and Prevention, using United States natality files, recently investigated state-specific changes in PTD rates among African Americans and whites from 50 states and the District of Columbia for the years 1990 and 1997. These data indicated that the PTD rate was twice as high among African Americans as among whites, although the disparity gap decreased as the result of an increase in preterm births among whites and a decrease among African Americans [16]. PTD was defined as a singleton, live birth occurring at 17 to 36 weeks' gestation. In 1990, the PTD rate among whites was 75.4 per 1000 live births (range: 56.6–103 live births), and 178.5 (range: 113.5–228.2 live births) among African Americans. In 1997, the PTD rate among whites increased to 83.7 (range: 65.4–106.7) and among African Americans it decreased 10% to 160.9 (range: 108.8–197.3). Although the PTD disparity in the United States has narrowed between African-American and whites nationally and in several states, the 1.5- to 2.4-fold excess risk for PTD among African Americans remains a public health concern if the 2010 national goal of eliminating PTD disparities among United States racial and ethnic groups is to be reached. Although the cause of PTD is unclear, it has been attributed to some known risk factors including maternal conditions, infection, stress, smoking, previous PTD, maternal age, and other demographic factors. Previous analyses have shown that change in maternal age distribution, time of entry into prenatal care, marital status, medical induction rates, and method of estimation of gestational age explained some, but not all, of the observed trends [16]. Although the higher risk for PTD among African Americans may reflect a greater prevalence or severity of these risk factors, and less access to health care and resources, these risk factors alone do not adequately account for the disparities. Two leading longitudinal models of health disparities [17] may provide a new context in which to evaluate the problem. The early programming model posits that exposures in early life could influence future reproductive potential. The cumulative pathways model conceptualizes a gradual decline in reproductive health resulting from cumulative wear and tear to the body's allostatic systems. Both are very worthy of consideration given the serious nature of the disparity and the recent knowledge that low birth weights, a very common sequelae of PTD, is associated with adult diseases, such as type 2 diabetes, hypertension, and coronary artery disease [18].

Prenatal care

Early and comprehensive prenatal care is the cornerstone of improving maternal perinatal outcomes. Women who receive delayed entry into prenatal care after the first 12 weeks of gestation, or no prenatal care, do not receive timely preventive care or education and are at risk for having undetected complications of pregnancy that can result in severe maternal or fetal morbidity, and sometimes death. In addition, these women are three times more likely to have a low–birth weight infant when compared with women who do receive early and comprehensive prenatal care [19]. Low–birth weight infants not only suffer from serious morbidities (eg, neurologic disorders, learning disabilities, delayed development, and so forth) but also contribute significantly to neonatal mortality rates in the United States. According to available national data, whereas 85% of white women begin their prenatal care in the first trimester, only 73% of African-American women do so [20]. Congress authorized the Medicaid extension program in the 1980s and it led to an increase in the number of pregnant women receiving prenatal care. Racial and ethnic disparities continue, however, and it is now known that the lack of money and health insurance are not the only major barriers to obtaining prenatal care. Others include lack of transportation, length of waiting time for care, lack of receptive providers, and poor access to specialty care.

Ovarian cancer

Although the incidence of ovarian cancer is lower among African-American women compared with white women, the relative survival of African-American women is poorer. The National Cancer database study [21] revealed that African-American women with advanced epithelial ovarian cancer were treated less aggressively than white women and were twice as likely not to receive appropriate medical therapy. Moreover, the prognostic disadvantage for African Americans persisted after controlling for African-American and white differences in age at diagnosis, household income, and type of treatment facility. In particular, African Americans diagnosed with advanced disease had poorer 5-year relative survival rates than whites treated at the same facility or other facilities, regardless of income level. More recently, in an analysis of members of a health maintenance organization with equal access to medical care, African-American women with ovarian cancer were found to have significantly higher death rates compared with white women, even after adjustment for stage, histology, and age at diagnosis [22]. The authors of the previously cited studies could not exclude differences in specialty of surgeon, extent of residual tumor, chemotherapy, and postoperative follow-up as possible prognostic influences. In an analysis of 38,012 patients with invasive epithelial ovarian cancer of six different race and ethnicities, as reported to the Surveillance, Epidemiology and End Results (SEER) Program of the National Cancer Institute, African Americans were more likely than whites to be diagnosed at older ages, with distant disease and with undifferentiated and unclassified cancers. After adjusting for age and stage at diagnosis and cancer histology, death rates were found to be significantly elevated among African Americans compared with whites [23]. In a separate study analyzing data from the SEER Program over a 30-year time period (1973–1997), the proportion of minorities diagnosed with epithelial ovarian cancer increased, and whereas overall survival of all patients continuously improved over time, older patients over 60 and African Americans continued to have the poorest survival [24].

Endometrial cancer

Survival rates following endometrial cancer diagnosis vary significantly between African-American and white women. Several factors are known to be associated with this disparity including higher stage and grade at presentation, worse histology, lower socioeconomic status, and greater clinical comorbidity. Most studies suggest, however, that substantial racial survival differences persist even after accounting for these factors. One explanation for the survival disparity may be differences in treatment. In a recent analysis of SEER data between 1992 and 1998, it was found that African-American women with endometrial cancer were significantly less likely to undergo primary surgery [25]. For instance, among patients with stage 1 disease, 7.7% of African-American women did not undergo surgery, whereas only 2.2% of white women did not undergo surgery. Similarly, among patients with stage 2 disease, 20.8% of African-American women did not undergo surgery compared with only 6% of white women. Racial differences in treatment were associated with racial differences in survival. These findings held true when the analysis was held constant for local-regional and metastatic disease. Furthermore, adjusting for differential use of surgery reduced the racial difference in survival for both subgroups, with the hazards ratio for the association between African-American race and mortality declining from 1.6 to 1.4 for women with local-regional disease and 1.7 to 1.5 for women with stage 4 disease. African-American women with endometrial cancer are less likely to undergo primary surgery and are more likely to die from their disease than are white women with endometrial cancer, all stages considered. These results corroborate the earlier findings in the seminal study by Hicks and coworkers [26] in which African-American women were less likely to undergo surgical therapy at all stages of disease. In addition, among surgically treated patients at advanced stages of disease, African Americans received adjuvant treatment less often and palliative chemotherapy more often than white patients. The lower rate of surgery for endometrial cancer among African-American women is supported by similar racial disparities in the use of surgery for many other conditions, including coronary artery bypass surgery, lung cancer resection, and renal transplantation [27–29].

Cervical cancer

Although invasive cervical cancer is theoretically a preventable disease, it causes tremendous morbidity and mortality among women of color in the United States, particularly African Americans. Some of the disparity is associated with lower rates of cervical cancer screening. For instance, in the National Breast and Cervical Cancer Early Detection Program study of low-income women, only 60% of 312,858 women reported ever having had a Pap smear [30]. Surprisingly, African Americans in some areas of the United States have higher Pap smear rates [31] but are still diagnosed in later stages of disease and have higher mortality rates than whites. One possible explanation for this is inadequate systems for follow-up of abnormal Pap smears and biopsies, delaying therapy. In addition, minority and underserved populations are frequently faced with limited availability of treatment options and may not have access to expert medical care. Another contributing factor is that of undertreatment as reflected in the study by Mundt and coworkers [32] in which fewer African Americans received intracavitary radiation than white patients. Interestingly, in this study, technical problems were cited to be more common in African Americans and the reason why they were less frequently treated with intracavitary therapy. Comorbid conditions protracted therapy more often in African Americans than whites, whereas poor compliance led to treatment interruptions in 28% of white patients in comparison with 10% of African Americans. Although poorer outcome was associated with lower hemoglobin levels at presentation and during treatment, no reason was given as to why African Americans received blood transfusions less often than whites. Minority women of low socioeconomic status tend to have comorbid diseases that contribute to poorer treatment outcomes for cervical cancer.

Summary

Until African Americans make a conscious decision to gain control of the social and economic context in which they live, and assume primary responsibility for their health, the reproductive disparities and associated deaths experienced by African-American women will persist. There is truly a need for continued clinical, epidemiologic, and molecular investigations into the problems. Ultimately, however, the permanent elimination of reproductive health disparities will require a social movement, led by members of the target population, informed by the findings of evidenced-based medicine, and fueled by a desire to raise the standard of living of the African-American community. As this occurs, all women will benefit.

References

[1] Kabir AA, Gabriella P, Steinmann WC, et al. Racial differences in cesareans: an analysis of US 2001 national inpatient sample data. Obstet Gynecol 2005;105:710.

[2] Abma J, Chandra A, Mosher W, et al. Fertility, family planning and women's health: new data from the 1995 National Survey of Family Growth. Vital Health Stat 23 1997;(19):1–114.

[3] Stephen E, Chandra A. Use of infertility services in the United States: 1995. Fam Plann Perspect 2000;32:132.

[4] Sharara FI, McClamrock HD. Differences in in-vitro fertilization (IVF) outcome between white and black women in an inner-city, university-based IVF program. Fertil Steril 2000;73: 1170.

[5] Grainger DA, et al. Racial disparity in clinical outcomes from women using advanced reproductive technologies (ART): analysis of 80,196 ART cycles from the SART database. Abstract No. O-93.

[6] Green JA, Robin JC, Scheiber M, et al. Racial and economic demographics of couples seeking infertility treatment. Am J Obstet Gynecol 2001;184:1080.

[7] Molock SD. Racial, cultural and religious issues in infertility counseling. In: Burns LH, Covington SN, editors. Infertility counseling: a comprehensive handbook for clinicians. New York: Parthenon; 1999.

[8] Sanders CJ. Surrogate motherhood and reproductive technologies: an African American perspective. Creigthton Law Rev 1992;25:1707.

[9] Peters KD, Kochanek KD, Murphy SL. Deaths: final data for 1996. National Vital Statistics Report, vol. 47, No. 9. Hyattsville (MD): US Department of Health and Human Services, CDC, National Center for Health Statistics; 1998.

[10] Ventura SJ, Martin JA, Curtin SC, et al. Report of final natality statistics, 1996. Monthly Vital Statistics Report, vol. 46, No. 11. Hyattsville (MD): US Department of Health and Human Services, CDC, National Center for Health Statistics; 1998.

[11] CDC. Maternal mortality—United States, 1982–1996. MMWR Morb Mortal Wkly Rep 1998;47:705.

[12] CDC. Differences in maternal mortality among black and white women—United States, 1990. MMWR Morb Mortal Wkly Rep 1995;44:6.

[13] Koonin L, MacKay A, Berg C, et al. Pregnancy-related mortality surveillance—United States, 1987–1990. MMWR Surveill Summ 1997;46:17–34.

[14] MacDorman MF, Atkinson JO. Infant mortality statistics from the period 1997 linked birth/ infant death data set. National Vital Statistics Report, vol. 47, No. 23. Hyattsville (MD): US Department of Health and Human Services, CDC, National Center for Health Statistics; 1999.

[15] Iyasu S, Becerra JE, Rowley DL, et al. Impact of very low birthweight on the black-white infant mortality gap. Am J Prev Med 1992;8:271.

[16] CDC. Preterm singleton births—United States, 1989–1996. MMWR 1999;48:185.

[17] Lu MC, Halfon N. Racial and ethnic disparities in birth outcomes: a life-course perspective. Matern Child Health J 2003;7:13.

[18] Sallout B, Walker M. The fetal origin of adult diseases. J Obstet Gynecol 2003;23:555.

[19] Healthy People 2000: national health promotion and disease prevention objectives. Washington: US Department of Health and Human Services, Public Health Service; 1998. DHHS publication 91–50213.

[20] Healthy people 2010. McClean (VA): International Medical Publishing; 2000.

[21] Parham G, Phillips JL, Hicks ML, et al. The National Cancer Data base report on malignant epithelial ovarian carcinoma in African-American women. Cancer 1997;80:816.

[22] McGuire V, Herrington L, Whittemore AS. Race, epithelial ovarian cancer survival and membership in a large health maintenance organization. Epidemiology 2002;13:231.

[23] McGuire V, Jesser CA, Whitemore AS. Survival among US women with invasive epithelial ovarian cancer. Gynecol Oncol 2002;84:399.

[24] Barnholtz-Sloan JS, Schwartz AG, et al. Ovarian cancer: changes in patterns at diagnosis and relative survival over the last three decades. Am J Obstet Gynecol 2003;189:1120.

[25] Randall TC, Armstrong K. Differences in treatment and outcome between African American and white women with endometrial cancer. J Clin Oncol 2003;21:4200.

[26] Hicks ML, Phillips JL, Parham G, et al. The National Cancer Data Base report on endometrial cancer in African American women. Cancer 2000;83:2629.

[27] Bach P, Cramer L, Warren J, et al. Racial differences in the treatment of early stage lung cancer. N Engl J Med 1999;341:1198.

[28] Daumit G, Hermann J, Coresh J, et al. use of cardiovascular procedures among black persons and white persons: a 7-year nationwide study in patients with renal disease. Ann Intern Med 1999;130:173.

[29] Eggers P. Racial differences in access to kidney transplantation. Health Care Financ Rev 1995;17:89.

[30] Lawson HW, Lee NC, Thames SF, et al. Cervical cancer screening among low income women. Results of a national screening program: 1991–1995. Obstet Gynecol 1998;92:74.

[31] Makuc DM, Freid VM, Kleinman JC. National trends in the use of preventive health care by women. Am J Public Health 1989;79:21.

[32] Mundt AJ, Connell PP, Campbell T, et al. Race and clinical outcome in patients with carcinoma of the uterine cervix treated with radiation therapy. Gynecol Oncol 1998;71:151.

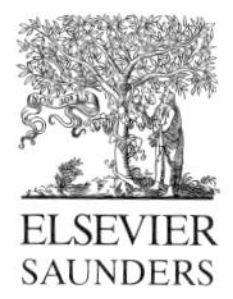

THE MEDICAL
CLINICS
OF NORTH AMERICA

Med Clin N Am 89 (2005) 945–948

Racial Disparities in Emergency Surgical Care

David C. Chang, PhD, MPH, MBA[a],
L.D. Britt, MD, MPH[b],*, Edward E. Cornwell, MD[a]

[a]Department of Surgery, Johns Hopkins School of Medicine, 600 North Wolfe Street,
#BLALOCK 688, Baltimore, MD 21287, USA
[b]Department of Surgery, Eastern Virginia Medical School, 825 Fairfax Avenue,
Suite 610, Norfolk, VA 23507, USA

The well-described race-based disparities in outcomes across a host of emergency surgical conditions have their genesis in several socioeconomic and physiologic factors. It is frequently difficult to quantify the relative contribution of socioeconomic factors because they are often closely related to stage of illness on presentation, aggressiveness of care, and comorbid medical conditions.

This article is devoted to medical/surgical emergency conditions that demonstrate race-based differences. These differences may not only have an impact on the ultimate outcome of care but may also have implications for the acute care practitioner in the emergency department.

Socioeconomic factors

Socioeconomic factors are often at play when race-based differences are observed in patient comorbid conditions facing the practitioner in acute care settings. For example, in a review of the emergency surgical care service at the Johns Hopkins Hospital, Weiss and colleagues found race-based differences in seroprevalence of hepatitis and HIV among a select group of 373 patients undergoing surgical procedures [1]. It was found that African American patients were more likely than whites to be seropositive for hepatitis B, hepatitis C, or HIV (42% versus 31%, $P < .05$) and for hepatitis C individually (38% versus 28%, $P < .05$). This disparity pales in

* Corresponding author.
E-mail address: brittld@evms.edu (L.D. Britt).

0025-7125/05/$ - see front matter © 2005 Elsevier Inc. All rights reserved.
doi:10.1016/j.mcna.2005.05.005   *medical.theclinics.com*

comparison to differences seen among patients with and without a history of intravenous drug abuse. There was a fivefold difference between intravenous drug abuse patients and non–intravenous drug abuse patients in their seroprevalence (71% versus 14%, $P < .05$); indeed, on multivariate analysis, race disappeared as a factor, whereas intravenous drug abuse persisted as a significant factor.

The report by Weiss and colleagues [1] is as much a description of the socioeconomically depressed neighborhood served by this university-based surgical service as it is a description of race-based disparity. To the extent that seroprevalence of hepatitis and HIV affect longevity, immunocompetence, and the ability to recover from surgical illness, any strategy designed to address this race-based disparity must consider socioeconomic factors.

Such factors were paramount in the configuration of a counseling program designed by the Trauma Service at the Johns Hopkins Hospital aimed at young (age 15–24 years) substance-abusing patients who survived a major injury (M. Yonas, D. Baker, E.E. Cornwell, MD, submitted for publication). Toxicology screens drawn on admission were used to identify young trauma patients who were using illicit drugs or abusing alcohol. These patients were offered counseling and assessed by a "Readiness to Change" interview tool. The group described in this study was disproportionately male (91%) and black (94%); however, their degree of socioeconomic disenfranchisement may be better represented by the fact that 63% were already high school dropouts and 71% had suffered penetrating injuries (gunshot or stab wounds) as opposed to blunt trauma. Although the initial assessment of attitudes regarding Readiness to Change among those patients experiencing penetrating injuries was encouraging, engaging patients in actual behavioral change was far more challenging, again demonstrating that social factors are largely at play in the barriers to overcoming race-based disparity in some emergency surgical conditions.

The social factors at play are further demonstrated by an assessment of the demographics of the community served by the previously referenced level 1 Trauma Center. Consider that the Trauma Center at Johns Hopkins Hospital sees a higher percentage of penetrating injuries (35%) among trauma admissions than any other trauma center in the state of Maryland, and that fully 80% of all trauma patients reside within a 5-mile radius of the hospital, a neighborhood that has a median household income that is two thirds of the state average [2]. Simply put, this hospital is located in a poor black neighborhood, and substance abuse disorders endemic in the neighborhood go a long way toward explaining several observed race-based disparities.

Physiologic differences

In a report by Chang and colleagues [3] that questioned the diagnostic value of the initial white blood cell count in trauma patients, an interesting race-based difference was parenthetically observed. Although there were no differences in outcomes, multiple linear regression analysis revealed that black trauma patients had significantly lower white blood cell counts on admission than their white counterparts. In view of earlier studies suggesting that the white blood cell count in healthy subjects is significantly lower in blacks than in whites, even after adjusting for the effects of sex, age, height, body mass index, alcohol use, and smoking, the presumption is that black patients begin with a lower preinjury white blood cell count [4,5]. This difference must be considered by the acute care practitioner evaluating patients suspected of having acute inflammatory conditions.

Health care access

Finally, health care access must be considered in race-based outcomes disparity. For example, a statewide database analysis by Dardik and colleagues [6] of nearly 10,000 patients undergoing carotid endarterectomy concluded that blacks had a higher in-hospital stroke rate and a longer length of stay than white patients. By way of explanation, the investigators found that performance of an operation by a "high-volume" surgeon was associated with a lower incidence of in-hospital stroke and that whites were more than twice as likely to have surgery performed by high-volume surgeons.

Similar methodology was employed in evaluating large statewide databases in finding that blacks were more likely to die when presenting with ruptured abdominal aortic aneurysms and more likely to receive an amputation when presenting with lower extremity peripheral vascular disease [7,8].

Access to health care may even play a role in racial disparities seen in the health of transplanted organs in renal transplant patients. In a report of 541 patients undergoing kidney transplants, Melancon and colleagues [9] found that black patients had a higher serum creatinine level than their white counterparts at 1 year and were more likely to have received the organs from cadavers (as opposed to living related donors).

These reports raise the strong suspicion that limited access to optimal surgical care may play a role in race-based outcome differences. Acute care practitioners are frequently the primary care providers responsible for referring patients who have symptoms suggestive of carotid stenosis to specialty care. In this regard, physicians must also honestly assess their own referring practices in attacking race-based disparities in outcomes.

Summary

Socioeconomic factors and differences in access to health care systems, perhaps more so than physiologic differences, play a significant role in race-based differences faced by acute care practitioners.

References

[1] Weiss ES, Makary MA, Wang T, et al. Prevalence of blood-borne pathogens in an urban, university-based general surgical practice. Ann Surg 2005;241(5):803–9.

[2] Chang D, Cornwell EE III, Phillips J, et al. Community characteristics and demographic information as determinants for a hospital-based injury prevention outreach program. Arch Surg 2003;138(12):1344–6.

[3] Chang DC, Cornwell EE III, Phillips J, et al. Early leukocytosis in trauma patients: what difference does it make? Curr Surg 2003;60(6):632–5.

[4] Reed WW, Diehl LF. Leukopenia, neutropenia, and reduced hemoglobin levels in healthy American blacks. Arch Intern Med 1991;151(3):501–5.

[5] Schwartz J, Weiss ST. Host and environmental factors influencing the peripheral blood leukocyte count. Am J Epidemiol 1991;134(12):1402–9.

[6] Dardik A, Bowman HM, Gordon TA, et al. Impact of race on the outcome of carotid endarterectomy: a population-based analysis of 9,842 recent elective procedures. Ann Surg 2000;232(5):704–9.

[7] Heller JA, Weinberg A, Arons R, et al. Two decades of abdominal aortic aneurysm repair: have we made any progress? J Vasc Surg 2000;32(6):1091–100.

[8] Dillingham TR, Pezzin LE, Mackenzie EJ. Racial differences in the incidence of limb loss secondary to peripheral vascular disease: a population-based study. Arch Phys Med Rehabil 2002;83(9):1252–7.

[9] Melancon J, Simpkins C, Cornwell EE, et al. Racial disparity in health of transplanted organs in renal transplant patients. Presented at the Society of Black Academic Surgeons. April 29, 2005.

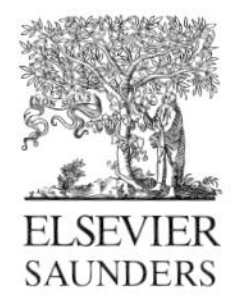

ELSEVIER
SAUNDERS

THE MEDICAL
CLINICS
OF NORTH AMERICA

Med Clin N Am 89 (2005) 949–975

Epidemiology of Type 2 Diabetes: Focus on Ethnic Minorities

Leonard E. Egede, MD, MS[a,b],
Samuel Dagogo-Jack, MD, FRCP[c,*]

[a]*Division of General Internal Medicine, Department of Medicine,
Medical University of South Carolina, 171 Ashley Avenue, Charleston, SC 29425, USA*
[b]*Ralph H. Johnson Veterans Affairs Medical Center, Charleston, SC, USA*
[c]*Division of Endocrinology, Diabetes, and Metabolism, Department of Medicine,
University of Tennessee Health Sciences Center, 951 Court Avenue, Room 335M, Memphis,
TN 38163, USA*

Diabetes mellitus is a chronic debilitating condition that affects approximately 18.2 million people or 6.3% of the United States population [1]. Diabetes is classified under four major categories [2]. Type 1 diabetes is characterized by beta cell destruction resulting in absolute insulin deficiency, occurs mostly in childhood, and accounts for 5% of all cases of diabetes. Type 2 diabetes is characterized predominantly by insulin resistance with relative insulin deficiency, occurs typically in adulthood, and accounts for 90% of all cases of diabetes. Gestational diabetes typically occurs during pregnancy, resolves postdelivery, and accounts for 3% of all cases of diabetes. A fourth category includes cases of diabetes that result from diverse etiologies and they account for about 2% of all cases of diabetes.

Prevalence and incidence of diabetes

The rate of diagnosed diabetes has grown steadily over time and is now approaching epidemic proportions. The age-adjusted prevalence rate of diagnosed diabetes increased from 2.77% in 1980 to 4.22% in 1999 [1]. There is also a similar trend in the rates of newly diagnosed cases of diabetes.

Dr. Egede is supported in part by grant no. 5K08HS11418 from the Agency for Health Care Research and Quality, Rockville, MD. Dr. Dagogo-Jack is supported in part by National Institutes of Health Clinical Research Center Grant no. MO1 RR00211.

* Corresponding author.
E-mail address: sdj@utmem.edu (S. Dagogo-Jack).

doi:10.1016/j.mcna.2005.03.004   *medical.theclinics.com*

Between 1980 and 1999 the incidence rate of diabetes increased from 0.23% to 0.34%. Currently, it is estimated that 1.3 million new cases of diabetes are diagnosed each year among people older than 20 years [1].

The prevalence of type 2 diabetes is higher in African Americans, Asian Americans and Pacific Islanders, Hispanic Americans, and Native Americans compared with whites. Current estimates show that there are 2.8 million African Americans who have diabetes, which represents 13% of the African-American population in the United States [3]. Diabetes in African Americans is more prevalent in women and in persons over 65 years of age. The prevalence of diabetes in African Americans has increased dramatically in recent times. Data from the National Health and Nutrition Examinations Survey showed that the prevalence of diabetes in African Americans doubled over a 12-year period with an increase from 8.9% in 1976 to 1980 to 18.2% in 1988 to 1994 [3]. Type 2 diabetes is the most prevalent type of diabetes in African Americans accounting for 90% to 95% of all cases, whereas type 1 diabetes accounts for 10% of the remainder [3]. Gestational diabetes is also highly prevalent in African Americans and several studies have shown that gestational diabetes is 50% to 80% more frequent in African-American women than in white women [3].

Prevalence of diabetes complications

Diabetes is a leading cause of cardiovascular disease, stroke, blindness, end-stage renal disease, and nontraumatic lower limb amputations [1]. Matched for age and sex, individuals who have diabetes have twofold to fourfold increased risk of cardiovascular disease–related deaths compared with people who do not have diabetes [1]. Diabetes accounts for 43% of all new cases of end-stage renal disease. Diabetes also accounts for 60% to 70% of cases of neuropathy and 60% of nontraumatic lower limb amputations in the United States [1]. In women, hyperglycemia is associated with spontaneous abortions in 15% to 20% of pregnancies and major birth defects in 5% to 10% of pregnancies [1].

Studies show that African Americans have higher incidence of and greater disability from diabetes complications than white Americans. Diabetes and hypertension, which are the two leading causes of end-stage renal disease, are more common in African Americans. African Americans who have diabetes are four times more likely to develop end-stage renal disease than their white counterparts who have diabetes [3]. Diabetic retinopathy is 40% to 50% more frequent in African Americans than in white Americans, which may be partly caused by the increased prevalence of hypertension in this group [3]. African Americans who have diabetes are much more likely to undergo a lower-extremity amputation than white or Hispanic Americans who have diabetes [3]. Studies have shown that death rates for people who have diabetes are 20% to 40% higher in African Americans compared with white Americans [3]. Evidence indicates that diabetes is a significant public health problem; however, African Americans seem disproportionately burdened with the complications and disability that result from poorly treated diabetes.

Risk factors for development of type 2 diabetes

Several large epidemiologic studies have identified risk factors for the development of type 2 diabetes [4]. These risk factors include belonging to an ethnic minority population, having a first-degree relative who has diabetes, obesity, living a sedentary lifestyle, age greater than 45 years, and having features of the metabolic syndrome (Box 1). The metabolic syndrome is associated with a significantly increased risk of developing diabetes and is characterized by the presence of three or more of the following risk factors (Table 1) [5]: abdominal obesity (waist circumference $>$ 102 cm in men and 88 cm in women); high serum triglycerides ($\geq$ 150 mg/dL); low high-density lipoprotein cholesterol ($<$ 40 mg/dL in men and $<$ 50 mg/dL in women); high blood pressure ($\geq$ 130/$\geq$ 85 mm Hg); and impaired fasting glucose ($\geq$ 110 mg/dL). The American Diabetes Association has subsequently revised normal fasting glucose as less than 100 mg/dL.

Box 1. Risks factors for type 2 diabetes

1. Age $\geq$ 45 years
2. Overweight (body mass index $\geq$ 25 kg/m^2)[a]
3. Family history of diabetes (ie, parents or siblings who have diabetes)
4. Habitual physical inactivity
5. Race or ethnicity (eg, African Americans, Hispanic Americans, Native Americans, Asian Americans, and Pacific Islanders)
6. Previously identified impaired fasting glucose or impaired glucose tolerance
7. History of gestational diabetes mellitus or delivery of baby weighing $>$ 9 lb
8. Hypertension ($\geq$ 140/90 mm Hg in adults)
9. High-density lipoprotein cholesterol $\leq$ 35 mg/dL (0.90 mmol/L) or a triglyceride level $\geq$ 250 mg/dL (2.82 mmol/L)
10. Polycystic ovary syndrome
11. History of vascular disease

---

[a] May not be correct for all ethnic groups.

Adapted from American Diabetes Association. Screening for type 2 diabetes. Diabetes Care 2004;27:S11–4; with permission.

Table 1
Clinical identification of the metabolic syndrome with three or more of the following risk factors

Risk factor	Defining level
Abdominal obesity (waist circumference)	
Men[a]	> 102 cm (> 40 in)
Women	> 88 cm (> 35 in)
Triglycerides	≥ 150 mg/dL
High-density lipoprotein cholesterol	
Men	< 40 mg/dL
Women	< 50 mg/dL
Blood pressure	≥ 130/≥ 85 mm Hg
Fasting glucose[b]	≥ 110 mg/dL

[a] 94–102 cm (37–40 in) in men predisposed to insulin resistance.

[b] Greater than or equal to 100 mg/dL based on new American Diabetes Association guidelines.

Adapted from Executive Summary of the Third Report of the National Cholesterol Education Program (NCEP) Expert Panel on Detection, Evaluation, and Treatment of High Blood Cholesterol in Adults (Adult Treatment Panel III). JAMA 2001;285:2486–97; with permission.

Etiology of ethnic disparity

There is some degree of uncertainty about the reasons for racial and ethnic differences in the prevalence and incidence of type 2 diabetes. It is thought that a combination of genetic factors and environmental triggers interact to confer an increased risk of diabetes in ethnic minorities.

Genetic factors

The thrifty gene hypothesis (Fig. 1) [6] explains type 2 diabetes, essential hypertension, and obesity as syndromes of impaired genetic homeostasis. This hypothesis posits that millions of years ago, human survival was dependent on genetically driven ability to ensure efficient storage of energy as fat. This metabolic thriftiness ensured survival during times of natural disasters. These "thrifty genes" have been transmitted over time even to the current era. Because famine and natural disasters no longer result in significant food shortages and humans are no longer as active as their primeval ancestors; these thrifty genes have essentially become a handicap. Thrifty genes in a new environment of guaranteed food supply and marked reduction in physical activity levels are now catalysts for the epidemic of obesity in affluent countries and among the elite in developing countries [7,8]. The thrifty gene hypothesis is generally accepted as a possible explanation for obesity, but its extension to explain type 2 diabetes has been challenged [9]. Unlike the case with obesity where thrifty genes possibly ensured survival by making available stored energy during starvation, diabetes reduces survival. The application of the thrifty gene hypothesis to type 2 diabetes seems not to be as convincing as its link to obesity.

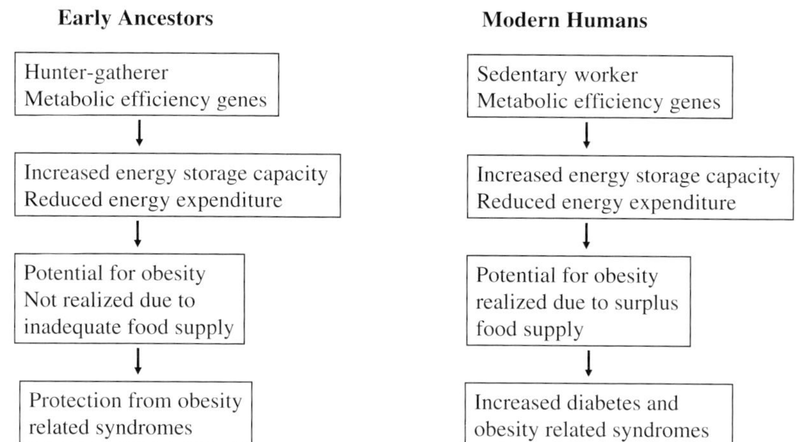

Fig. 1. Schema for the thrifty gene hypothesis. (*Adapted from* Dagogo-Jack S. Ethnic disparities in type 2 diabetes: pathophysiology and implications for prevention and management. J Natl Med Assoc 2003;95:774–89; with permission.)

Alternative hypotheses

One alternative hypothesis is called "antagonistic pleiotropy" [10]. This concept suggests that there might be a tradeoff between fitness components in earlier and later stages of life. It postulates that thriftiness at a younger age ensures survival and reproductive viability, but after middle age, thrifty genes predispose to diabetes. The major weakness of antagonistic pleiotropy is that it lacks empirical examples in nature. The second alternative is the "genetic trash can" hypothesis. This hypothesis postulates that there is conservation of multiple, individually neutral gene mutations that confer aggregate risks for type 2 diabetes occur over time. The accumulation and concentration of these diabetogenes in a given population leads to increased prevalence of type 2 diabetes [9,11]. Because diabetogenes are generally recessive, it is expected that ethnic populations that are typically less exogamous than European populations have an increased prevalence of type 2 diabetes [9]. Exogamy, migrations, conquests, invasions, interbreeding, and admixtures exert a dilutional effect on mutant genes. For example, many aboriginal societies have experienced less of these diluting events than have whites and tend to have higher prevalence of diabetes [9,12,13]. These diabetogenes may partially explain the increased prevalence of type 2 diabetes in ethnic minorities.

Environmental triggers

The environment plays an important role in uncovering latent genetic predispositions [14]. This was clearly demonstrated in studies of Japanese immigrants to the United States that showed a threefold increase in the rate of type 2 diabetes compared with native Japanese [15]. In the Japanese immigrants, environmental triggers, including changes in diet and lifestyle, most probably accounted for the expression of the innate genetic predisposition to type 2 diabetes because such dramatic increase in disease prevalence in humans cannot be attributed to sudden new genetic mutations.

The exact mechanisms whereby environmental triggers induce diabetes in genetically predisposed persons are not known with certainty. Ethnic differences in diabetes risk factors alone, however, cannot account for the marked disparities in diabetes prevalence. For example, although obesity is the single most compelling (and most predictable) risk factor for type 2 diabetes in the general population [16], the incidence of diabetes among even massively obese persons is not 100%. Indeed, obesity triggers diabetes only in a susceptible minority. Nonetheless, because obesity is more prevalent among African-American and Hispanic subjects compared with whites at the time of diagnosis of type 2 diabetes [16,17], it is possible that individual risk factors may exert differential effects on diabetes risk among the different ethnic groups.

The metabolic syndrome

The risk factors for impaired fasting glucose (IGT) and type 2 diabetes overlap considerably, with insulin resistance as a common underlying thread. Many patients who have IGT have features of the insulin-resistance (metabolic) syndrome, including decreased high-density lipoprotein cholesterol levels; increased low-density lipoprotein cholesterol levels (particularly small, dense low-density lipoprotein particles); hypertriglyceridemia; upper body obesity; hyperinsulinemia; hypertension; and abnormal fibrinolysis.

The metabolic syndrome (see Table 1) [5] affects millions of prediabetic persons in the United States and is associated with a twofold increased risk for cardiovascular disease. At present, no drug therapy has been approved for treatment of prediabetic persons who have the metabolic syndrome. Lifestyle modifications (caloric restriction, reduction in saturated fats, increased physical activity) are remarkably effective, however, in preventing progression to diabetes and improving cardiovascular disease risk markers [18].

Pathophysiology of type 2 diabetes

Type 2 diabetes is characterized by impaired insulin action (insulin resistance) and impaired pancreatic beta cell function. Insulin resistance occurs when there is reduced sensitivity in body tissues to the action of insulin [19]. Over time higher concentrations of insulin are required to stimulate glucose disposal in peripheral tissues and suppress glucose production in the liver [19]. Eventually, functional defects in the pancreatic beta cells prevent adequate insulin production in response to the high demands in the peripheral tissues resulting in overt type 2 diabetes (Fig. 2). Insulin resistance also contributes to other defects that are seen in type 2 diabetes including dyslipidemia, hypertension, and increased cardiovascular risk [19].

Underlying pathophysiology in ethnic minorities

In ethnic minority groups, the concurrent role of insulin resistance and beta cell dysfunction in predicting the development of type 2 diabetes was confirmed in a longitudinal study of Pima Indians [20]. Studies that compared various populations of West African descendants (including African Americans and native Ghanaians) and whites have reported higher degrees of insulin resistance among West African descendants [21,22]. These studies have also suggested alterations in hepatic insulin clearance in African populations compared with whites [21]. The Insulin Resistance Atherosclerosis Study also showed higher degrees of insulin resistance among African Americans and Hispanics than whites [23]. The ethnic differences in insulin

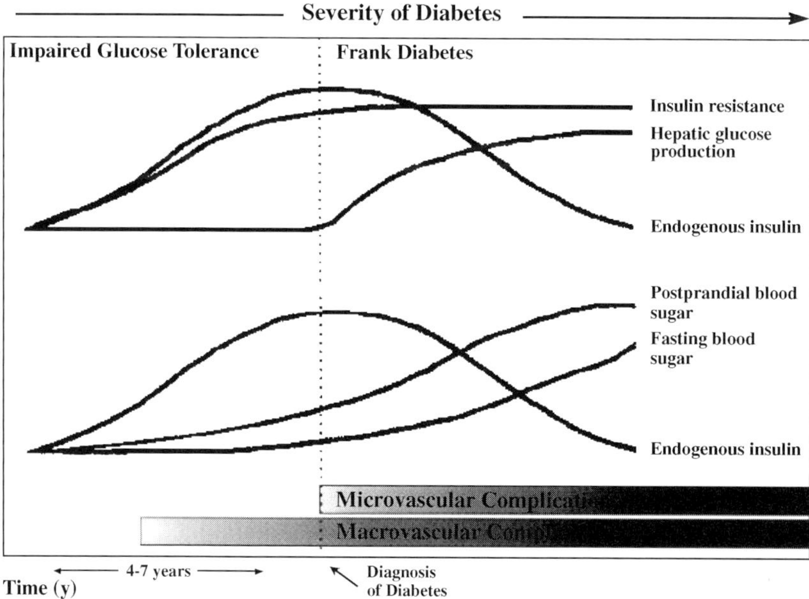

Fig. 2. Natural history of type 2 diabetes. The prediabetic state of impaired glucose tolerance is characterized by increasing insulin resistance, compensatory hyperinsulinemia, and mild postprandial hyperglycemia. Initially, fasting blood glucose levels are maintained in near normal ranges. The beta cell then begins to fail, resulting in higher postprandial glucose levels and, with further loss of insulin secretory capacity and impaired glucorecognition, fasting blood glucose and hepatic glucose production increase. (*Adapted from* Ramlo-Halstead. The natural history of type 2 diabetes. Implications for clinical practice. Prim Care 1999;26:771–89; with permission.)

sensitivity persisted after adjusting for age, gender, clinic site, body mass index, waist-to-hip ratio, and physical activity score [23]. These studies provide evidence for genetically driven insulin resistance as an underlying factor for the ethnic disparities in the prevalence of type 2 diabetes.

Recent findings from the Diabetes Prevention Program [18] offer interesting new perspectives: the incidence of type 2 diabetes was found to be similar (approximately 11%) among African Americans, Asian Americans and Pacific Islanders, white Americans, Hispanic Americans, and Native Americans. The well-known ethnic disparity in the risk for type 2 diabetes was surprisingly not evident among the Diabetes Prevention Program cohort of approximately 3000 subjects who have IGT, who were followed for 2 to 4 years. By definition, persons who have IGT have normal fasting plasma glucose levels and 2-hour levels of 140 to 199 mg/dL during a 75-g oral glucose tolerance test. The finding of similar rates of diabetes across racial or ethnic groups in the Diabetes Prevention Program suggests that once individuals have progressed from normal glucose tolerance to IGT, the risk of further progression to diabetes is the same across ethnic groups. The ethnic or genetic factors that predispose to diabetes must have exerted their maximal effects during the transition from normal metabolism to IGT. This intriguing and novel notion has obvious implications for the design and translation of primary prevention strategies.

Mechanisms and mediators of diabetes complications

Theoretically, the increased microvascular complications of diabetes among ethnic minorities may be caused by primary (genetic) susceptibility or secondary (acquired) factors.

Primary or genetic susceptibility

There is some evidence for familial clustering of microvascular complications, especially diabetic nephropathy, in certain ethnic minority populations [24]. This suggests a role for hereditary factors in the pathogenesis of microvascular complications. Data from landmark studies offer an expanded perspective in this area. In the Diabetes Control and Complications Trial [25], intensive glycemic control resulted in a 50% to 70% reduction in the risk of development of retinopathy, neuropathy, or nephropathy. In the United Kingdom Prospective Diabetes Study (UKPDS) [26], intensive glucose control reduced the risk of a doubling of serum creatinine by 74%, among other benefits. These rather large effects of glycemic control on target organ end points indicate that genetic factors are permissive rather than obligate determinants of risk. In the National Health and Nutrition Examinations Survey III retinopathy data [27], the African-American–white disparity no longer was significant after adjusting for known risk factors for retinopathy, such as chronicity of diabetes, hemoglobin A_{1c} level, and blood pressure.

Secondary or acquired factors

Nongenetic factors that could explain the development of complications of diabetes include patient factors, suboptimal quality of care, and socioeconomic factors.

Patient adherence

Physicians and other health care providers often explain away suboptimal outcome on the basis of possible nonadherence to therapeutic recommendations. Yet careful studies have revealed no evidence of significant ethnic or racial differences in global compliance with diabetes-related tasks (Table 2) [28]. Similarly, a recent study did not find significant racial or ethnic differences in adherence to medications and dietary or exercise recommendations [29]. A notable exception is self-monitoring of blood glucose (SMBG), where approximately 18% of African-American patients were testing at the minimal recommended frequency compared with approximately 30% of Hispanic and white patients [30]. It must be noted, however, that the frequency of self-monitoring is suboptimal even among Hispanics and whites.

A casual impression of general nonadherence tends to undermine dedicated therapeutic action by health care providers, which could be tragic for the effective management of diabetes. It must be stressed that a positive interaction between patients and physicians is a critical element of successful management of chronic disorders. It is imperative that the label of nonadherence be avoided, unless admitted to by patients or proved by objective criteria. Even after a patient has been found to be nonadherent, it behooves the caregiver to understand and attempt to correct the barriers or misguided premise that led to such behavior.

Socioeconomic factors

There is abundant literature on the contributions of low socioeconomic status, limitations in access to care, lack of health insurance or under-insurance, and other socioeconomic barriers to increased burden of diabetes and its complications [31,32]. One worrisome example is diabetic ketoacidosis: in one study of African Americans, cessation of insulin was the major precipitating cause of diabetic ketoacidosis [33]. It was further documented in that study that 43% of patients stopped taking insulin because they had no means to replenish their spent stock of insulin and 25% stopped because of a fundamental misunderstanding of the role of insulin therapy during sick days [33]. Nearly two thirds of the cases of diabetic ketoacidosis among African Americans in that study were preventable, either through renewal of insulin supplies or education to improve self-management skills.

Indeed, much of what passes as ethnic disparities in clinical outcomes may be mediated to a large extent by socioeconomic factors. For example,

Table 2
Diabetes management: patient compliance and practices by ethnicity

| | Ethnicity (%) | | |
Patient compliance and practices	Hispanic	African-American	White
Missed clinic	1.4	1.9	1.5
Noncompliance	34.0	27.0	26.0
Alcoholism	3.4	2.2	2.5
Missed foot clinic	0.0	2.7	5.6
Missed weight visit	17.0	15.0	9.0
Missed eye clinic	0.0	2.0	7.0

There were no significant racial/ethnic differences in compliance behavior.

Adapted from Martin TI, Selby JV, Zhang D. Physician and patient preventive practices in NIDDM in a large urban managed-care organization. Diabetes Care 1995;18:1124–32; with permission.

the marked ethnic disparity in lower extremity amputation rates observed in the general diabetic population is not evident in an ethnically diverse population with uniform health care coverage [34]. Even the low frequency of SMBG has socioeconomic underpinnings: with identical health insurance coverage, the frequency of SMBG among African Americans increased to match or exceed that of Asian, Hispanic, or white patients [34].

Physician practices

Another possible explanation for the increased morbidity from diabetes in ethnic minorities is systematic delivery of suboptimal care. Saadine et al [35] used two nationally representative surveys to document the quality of diabetes care during 1988 to 1995 and they found significant gaps between recommended diabetes care and the care patients actually received (Table 3). This study, which provides a national benchmark for the quality of diabetes care, found that 18% of participants had poor glycemic control (hemoglobin $A_{1c} > 9.5\%$); 34% had poorly controlled blood pressure ($> 140/90$ mm Hg); 58% had poorly controlled low-density lipoprotein cholesterol (> 130 mg/dL); and up to 15% of participants did not have recommended biannual cholesterol measurements. In addition, 37% of participants did not have a dilated eye examination, and 45% did not have a foot examination. After controlling for age, sex, ethnicity, education level, insulin use, and duration of diabetes, non-Hispanic African Americans who have diabetes were more likely to have poor glycemic control and poorly controlled blood pressures (Table 4).

Other studies have shown that African Americans who have diabetes are less likely to receive recommended influenza and pneumonia vaccinations despite repeated visits to primary care physicians [36–38]. Such reports indicate that there are disparities in the quality of care rendered to persons who have diabetes. National surveys do not support the notion of widespread, systematic undertreatment of minority patients, however, as

Table 3
Persons aged 18 to 75 who have diabetes in the Third US National Health and Nutrition Examination Survey and the Behavioral Risk Factors Surveillance System receiving preventive care

DQIP indicators	Patients % (95% CI)
Accountability measures	
$\geq$ 1 test for hemoglobin A_{1c}/y	28.8 (25.1–32.5)
Hemoglobin A_{1c} level $>$ 9.5%	18.0 (15.7–22.3)
Biannual lipid profile	85.3 (83.1–88.6)
LDL cholesterol level $<$ 3.4 mmol/L ($<$ 130 mg/dL)	42.0 (34.9–49.1)
Blood pressure $<$ 140/90 mm Hg	65.7 (62.0–69.4)
Annual dilated eye examination	63.3 (59.6–67.0)
Annual foot examination	54.8 (51.3–58.3)
Quality improvement measures	
Hemoglobin A_{1c} level (%)	
$<$ 7.0	42.9 (37.5–48.4)
7.0–7.9	15.7 (12.6–18.8)
8.0–8.9	16.4 (11.7–21.1)
9.0–9.9	10.0 (7.6–12.4)
$\geq$ 10.0	14.9 (11.6–18.2)
LDL cholesterol level	
$<$ 2.6 mmol/L ($<$ 100 mg/dL)	11.0 (5.9–16.1)
2.6–3.3 mmol/L (100–129 mg/dL)	31.1 (23.1–39.1)
3.4–4.1 mmol/L (130–159 mg/dL)	34.4 (26.0–42.8)
$>$ 4.2 mmol/L ($>$ 160 mg/dL)	23.6 (16.2–31.0)
Systolic blood pressure (mm Hg)	
$<$ 140	68.5 (65.4–71.6)
140–159	21.1 (17.4–24.8)
160–179	9.1 (6.4–11.8)
180–209	1.3 (0.5–2.1)
$>$ 210	0
Diastolic blood pressure (mm Hg)	
$<$ 90	93.5 (91.0–96.1)
90–99	5.5 (3.1–7.9)
100–109	0.9 (0.1–1.7)
110–119	0.1 (0.02–0.22)
$>$ 120	0
Other quality-of-care measures[a]	
Annual influenza vaccine	45.7 (42.4–47.0)
Pneumococcal vaccine	26.5 (23.2–29.8)
Self-monitoring blood glucose test (at least once daily)	38.0 (34.5–41.5)
Annual dental examination	58.0 (52.3–63.7)

Abbreviations: DQIP, Diabetes Quality Improvement Project; LDL, low density lipoprotein.
[a] Not currently part of the standard DQIP measures of care.
Adapted from Saaddine JB, Engelgau MM, Beckles GL, et al. A diabetes report card for the United States: quality of care in the 1990s. Ann Intern Med 2002;136:565–74; with permission.

an explanation for the increased morbidity from diabetes [39]. There is no evidence of discrimination in referral patterns or use of insulin or oral agents for correction of hyperglycemia [39]. What is evident is a poor overall state of diabetes control in the nation at large [35,40,41].

Table 4
Predictive marginal prevalence of accountability measures for persons in the Third US National Health and Nutritional Examination Survey and the Behavioral Risk Factors Surveillance System according to demographic and clinical variables

Criteria	Ethnicity % (95% CI)		
	Non-Hispanic white	Non-Hispanic African-American	Hispanic- or Mexican-American
Hemoglobin A$_{1c}$ level > 9.5% (n = 877)	15.9 (12.0–19.8)*	27.1 (21.2–33.0)*	22.2 (14.4–30.0)
Biannual lipid test (n = 2630)	85.2 (83.7–87.7)	83.6 (77.7–89.5)	85.6 (78.1–93.7)
LDL cholesterol level < 130 mg/dL (n = 271)	37.1 (29.3–44.9)	40.2 (24.5–55.9)	53.7 (38.0–69.4)
Blood pressure < 140/90 mm Hg (n = 877)	64.8 (58.9–70.7)*	56.6 (48.8–64.4)*	64.1 (58.2–70.0)
Annual dilated eye examination (n = 2630)	63.3 (59.4–67.2)	68.6 (60.8–76.4)	60.7 (47.0–74.4)
Annual foot examination (n = 2567)	53.7 (49.8–57.6)	59.2 (49.4–69.0)	60.7 (48.9–72.5)

* $P < 0.05$ for the difference.

Adapted from Saaddine JB, Engelgau MM, Beckles GL, et al. A diabetes report card for the United States: quality of care in the 1990s. Ann Intern Med 2002;136:565–74; with permission.

Cost of treating diabetes

Several studies have shown that diabetes imposes substantial economic burden on both the individual and society. One of the early studies on the economic burden of diabetes was conducted in 1986 [42]. It showed that the total cost of non–insulin dependent diabetes (type 2 diabetes) was $11.6 billion, of which $6.8 billion was caused by direct medical cost. Another study used data from the 1996 Medical Expenditures Survey to calculate the economic burden of five chronic conditions [43]. The results of that study showed that total health costs for treating diabetes was $57.6 billion. A third study was the one sponsored by the American Diabetes Association [44], which found that total cost of diabetes in 1997 was $98 billion. The study found that $44 of the $98 billion resulted from direct medical costs, whereas $54 billion was caused by indirect costs including disability, work loss, and premature mortality. Recent estimates of medical expenditures in the United States in 2002 [45] show that direct and indirect medical expenditures attributable to diabetes totaled $132 billion. Approximately $91.8 billion was attributable to direct medical care for diabetes.

Cost effectiveness of treatments for diabetes

The UKPDS is the largest study to date on the effectiveness of treatment for type 2 diabetes. The UKPDS was a multicenter, prospective, randomized, intervention trial of approximately 5100 newly diagnosed patients who have type 2 diabetes aimed to determine whether improved blood glucose control prevents complications and reduces associated morbidity and mortality [46]. The planned median follow-up was 9 years (range 3–16 years). Intensive blood-glucose control by either sulfonylureas or insulin substantially decreased the risk of microvascular complications, but not macrovascular disease [26].

The cost-effectiveness study that accompanied the UKPDS found that intensive blood glucose control in patients who have type 2 diabetes significantly increased treatment costs but substantially reduced the cost of complications and increased the time free of complications [47]. Intensive glucose control increased treatment costs by £695 per patient but reduced the cost of complications by £957 compared with conventional treatment and the incremental cost per event-free year gained ranged from £563 to £1166.

Recently, a cost effectiveness study of intensive glycemic control for type 2 diabetes was conducted in the United States [48]. The study modeled a hypothetical cohort of individuals living in the United States aged 25 years or older, who were newly diagnosed with type 2 diabetes. The incremental cost-effectiveness ratio for intensive glycemic control was $41,384 per quality-adjusted life year. This ratio increased from $9614 per quality-adjusted life year in patients aged 25 to 34 years to $2.1 million per quality-adjusted life year for patients aged 85 to 94 years. These studies show that intensive glycemic control improves health outcomes and the cost-effectiveness ratio for intensive glycemic control is comparable with those of other frequently adopted health care interventions.

Treatments for type 2 diabetes

Studies have shown that when blood glucose levels are controlled to a similar degree, the rates of diabetic nephropathy, neuropathy, and retinopathy are similar in white and nonwhite patients. In the recently concluded Diabetes Prevention Study, the response rates to intensive lifestyle or pharmacologic intervention were identical in African Americans, Asian Americans and Pacific Islanders, Hispanics, Native Americans, and white Americans [18]. These findings, demonstrating lack of ethnic disparity in the responsiveness to antidiabetic regimen, are indeed heartening. The targets for glycemic control for persons who have diabetes, as recommended by the American Diabetes Association [49], are average preprandial blood glucose values of 90 to 130 mg/dL; peak postprandial blood glucose values of less than 180 mg/dL; and hemoglobin A_{1c} 7% or lower. The American College of Endocrinology Diabetes Mellitus Consensus Conference recommends a fasting glucose target of less than 110 mg/dL and a hemoglobin A_{1c} of less than 6.5% [50]. All recommendations are in general agreement that the goals of diabetes management are normalization or near-normalization of fasting and postprandial blood glucose levels and prevention of acute and long-term complications.

Nonpharmacologic approaches

Self-monitoring of home blood glucose

SMBG is an important (but underused) tool of diabetes management and education. Performance of SMBG is associated with superior glycemic control [51]. The recommended frequency of SMBG is two to four times daily for insulin-treated patients. The optimal frequency has not been established for patients who have type 2 diabetes treated with oral agents, but regular SMBG (at least once daily) is recommended [49]. The physician should review the results of SMBG and give appropriate feedback.

Diabetes education and counseling

Diabetes education and dietary and exercise counseling are effective in minority populations [52] and these approaches should be promoted as important adjuncts to pharmacotherapy of type 2 diabetes. This is best accomplished through referral to certified diabetes educators and dietitians. Regular physical activity enhances insulin sensitivity, decreases abdominal obesity, and improves blood pressure and lipid levels. Exercise programs should be tailored to individual patients' physical condition, and should always include warm-up and cool-down periods. To be effective, programs should use aerobic exercise (eg, walking, cycling, swimming) at approximately 60% of maximum oxygen use for 30 minutes, three or more times per week. Cardiac screening with stress electrocardiogram is recommended for patients aged 35 years or older, especially those who have been sedentary.

Lifestyle modification

Genetically driven insulin resistance is an underlying feature of type 2 diabetes in minority populations. Given this backdrop, it can be predicted that interventions that improve insulin sensitivity will be particularly effective in these populations. Indeed, experience with lifestyle interventions supports such a notion. Restriction of total and saturated fat intake, with augmentation of complex carbohydrates and dietary fiber, enhances insulin sensitivity [53]. Using a dietary approach based broadly on these principles, Ziemer et al [52] demonstrated excellent response rates among African-American patients who have type 2 diabetes. Following 6 to 12 months of initiation of the program, hemoglobin A_{1c} levels decreased by nearly 2% and the need for insulin secretogogues and exogenous insulin was substantially reduced [52]. The basis for the improved glycemic control is most consistent with amelioration of insulin resistance. Regular exercise, caloric restriction, and weight loss have profound insulin-sensitizing effects that constitute a prophylaxis against the development of diabetes in high-risk patients, as was shown in the Diabetes Prevention Program [18].

Pharmacologic approaches

The ideal treatment for type 2 diabetes should reverse insulin resistance (and the associated metabolic syndrome); normalize hepatic glucose production; improve beta cell function; and prevent the development of long-term complications [54]. Aggressive glycemic control is needed to maintain hemoglobin A_{1c} levels below 6.5% and to prevent the development of diabetic complications [50]. Medications used for treating diabetes include insulin and oral agents. Pharmacotherapy for diabetes is most effective if initiated as part of a comprehensive management plan that includes SMBG, patient education, and dietary and exercise counseling. The mnemonic MEDEM (_m_onitoring, _e_ducation, _d_iet, _e_xercise, _m_edications) can be used to recall the key modalities of diabetes management [55].

The agents currently approved for oral therapy of type 2 diabetes belong to five distinct chemical classes (Table 5). Functionally, these agents can be classified into insulin secretogogues (sulfonylureas, repaglinide, and nateglinide); insulin sensitizers (biguanides, thiazolidinediones [TZDs]); and α-glucosidase inhibitors (acarbose and miglitol). All of these agents have tissue-specific actions to improve blood glucose control. The initial choice of medication for control of hyperglycemia in type 2 diabetes patients is a matter of clinical judgment. Monotherapy with maximum doses of insulin secretogogues, metformin, or TZDs yields comparable glucose-lowering effects [54,56]. An additional basis for selecting oral agents relates to their nonglycemic effects, especially those that impact on cardiovascular risk factors. Aggressive control of hypertension, dyslipidemia, and obesity should be integrated into routine diabetes management practices.

Insulin secretogogues

Insulin secretogogues exert their glucose-lowering effects acutely, whereas the maximum effects of metformin or TZDs may not be observed until after several weeks of medication. Because residual pancreatic beta cell function is required for the glucose-lowering effects of all insulin secretogogues, metformin, and TZDs, many patients who have advanced type 2 diabetes do not respond satisfactorily to any of these agents. Insulin therapy may be an early choice for such patients. Moreover, the toxicity profile of a given oral agent may preclude its use in patients who have comorbid conditions.

α-Glucosidase inhibitors

The α-glucosidase inhibitors (acarbose, miglitol) are less potent in monotherapy, but are useful options for combination therapy.

Thiazolidinediones

Of the numerous classes of medication available for treatment of type 2 diabetes, only the TZDs exploit tissue sensitization to insulin as their

Table 5
Oral agents for the treatment of type 2 diabetes mellitus

Class/generic name	Trade name	Dose range (mg/d)
Single agents		
Sulfonylureas		
Acetohexamide	Dymelor	250–1500
Tolazamide	Tolinase	100–750
Tolbutamide	Orinase	100–750
Chlorpropamide	Diabinese	100–750
Glipizide	Glucotrol	5–40
Glipizide extended release	Glucotrol XL	5–20
Glyburide	Micronase	1.25–20
	Diaβeta	1.25–20
Glyburide, micronized	Glynase	1.5–12
Glimepiride	Amaryl	1–8
Secretagogues		
Repaglinide	Prandin	1–16
Nateglinide	Starlix	120–360
α-Glucosidase inhibitors		
Acarbose	Precose	25–300
Miglitol	Glyset	25–300
Biguanides		
Metformin	Glucophage	850–2550
Metformin, extended release	Glucophage XR	500–2000
Thiazolidinediones		
Rosiglitazone	Avandia	4–8
Pioglitazone	Actos	15–45
Combination agents		
Metformin + glipizide	Metaglip	2.5/250–20/2000
Metformin + glyburide	Glucovance	2.5/250–20/2000
Metformin + rosiglitazone	Avandamet	2/500–8/2000

dominant mechanism of action [57]. Rosiglitazone and pioglitazone are the two TZDs in current clinical use. The TZDs enhance insulin sensitivity by mechanisms that involve binding to a nuclear receptor (called peroxisome proliferator-activated receptor γ). Interaction between TZDs and peroxisome proliferator-activated receptor γ influences the transcription of genes that regulate carbohydrate and lipid metabolism.

The TZDs have beneficial effects on many components of the metabolic syndrome, thereby improving risk markers for cardiovascular disease [58]. There is also evidence that the TZDs exert a favorable effect on pancreatic beta cell function [59,60]. A dual effect on insulin resistance and beta cell function by the TZDs can be expected to result in improved glycemic control that is sustained over long periods [61], thereby reducing the risk for diabetic complications. As predicted, exquisite sensitivity to the metabolic effects of rosiglitazone has been reported in ethnic minority populations, including African Americans, Mexican Americans, and Chinese patients, who have type 2 diabetes [60,62,63].

The adverse effects of the TZD class include weight gain and edema from fluid retention. The weight can be minimized by caloric restriction and physical activity. Edema is uncommon ($< 5\%$) during TZD monotherapy but can occur in up to approximately 15% of persons treated with TZDs in combination with insulin or insulin secretogogues. Plasma volume expansion is a class effect of the TZDs and only in a small minority ($< 1\%$) of patients treated with TZDs is the edema associated with congestive heart failure [64]. Because increased plasma volume is undesirable in the setting of pre-existing cardiac congestion, use of TZDs is not appropriate in patients who have New York Heart Association class III or IV congestive heart failure [64]. Baseline and periodical liver function testing is required in patients treated with TZD; alanine transaminase levels greater than 2.5 times the upper normal limit preclude the use of these agents.

Early combination therapy

The UKPDS showed the futility of monotherapy as a strategy for long-term glycemic control in type 2 diabetes [65]. After 3 years, only about 50% of patients enrolled in the UKPDS were able to maintain the hemoglobin A_{1c} goal of 7% or lower, and by 9 years, the number had declined to about 25%. This loss of glycemic control is attributable to the fact that the traditional antidiabetic agents (sulfonylureas, metformin, insulin) do not preserve beta cell function or directly impact insulin resistance, two core defects underlying type 2 diabetes. Early use of drug combinations is the rationale approach to sustained glycemic control and prevention of complications in patients who have type 2 diabetes. Because of the longer latency of disease in minority populations with a high burden of undiagnosed diabetes [66], early use of combination therapy should be considered in these populations. Medications for combination therapy should be selected from drug classes that lower blood glucose by different mechanisms, to ensure additive or synergistic effects and to maximize nonglycemic benefits.

Each of the available antidiabetic drugs has been documented to be a suitable agent for use in combination with drugs from other classes. Perhaps the best-documented treatment strategy is one that combines an insulin sensitizer agent with a secretogogue. The use of two sensitizer drugs, such as a TZD and metformin, is an effective strategy that improves glycemic control while minimizing the risks of weight gain and hypoglycemia [67–69].

Indeed, double sensitizer therapy has particular merit among high-risk ethnic populations with endemic insulin resistance. The recent introduction of fixed-dose combination agents facilitates the practice of combination therapy. Theoretically, use of these fixed-dose agents may augur well for long-term medication compliance in diabetes patients, who often also take several medications for comorbid conditions. Currently, there are three such fixed-dose combination agents: (1) glyburide-metformin (Glucovance; Bristol-Myers Squibb, Princeton, New Jersey); (2) rosiglitazone-metformin (Avandamet; GlaxoSmithKline, Research Triangle Park, North Carolina); and (3) metformin-glipizide (Metaglip; Bristol-Myers Squibb). Other fixed-dose combinations are in development. In using these fixed-dose combination products, care must be taken to ensure that patients meet the safety criteria for use of each individual component.

Combination therapy is most effective if initiated as part of a comprehensive diabetes care plan, and after a careful consideration of possible barriers to metabolic control. The decision to continue a combination regimen should be based on evidence of continuing efficacy, safety, and tolerability and such evidence should be re-evaluated at frequent intervals. The efficacy of most combination regimens can be reliably evaluated over a 3- to 6-month period. Patients who have been on an oral drug combination regimen for 3 to 6 months and still have hemoglobin A_{1c} that exceeds 7% may be candidates for supplemental insulin therapy.

Indications for insulin therapy in type 2 diabetes

In the UKPDS, estimates of pancreatic beta-cell function revealed that in most patients who have type 2 diabetes beta-cell function had decreased by about 50% at the time of diagnosis and continued to deteriorate over time [70]. The progressive decline in beta-cell function predicts a future need for exogenous insulin in type 2 diabetes patients. Immediate insulin therapy is indicated for initial stabilization of type 2 diabetes patients who have ketoacidosis, hyperosmolar state, or severe hyperglycemia. In otherwise stable patients, exogenous insulin can be considered as an adjunct to oral agents if glycemic control is suboptimal. Insulin therapy can be initiated in a number of ways.

Patients who have type 2 diabetes managed with oral agents for many years are understandably reticent about the prospects of starting insulin. Care must be taken to explain the rationale and benefits of optimizing glycemic control and the demonstrated efficacy of insulin in accomplishing that objective. The physician may also need to address the exaggerated and often inaccurate concerns that some patients harbor regarding the safety of insulin. Preemptive discussion of the phenomenon of "pseudohypoglycemia" may also help to increase the patient's confidence in the period following initiation of insulin therapy. Subjective symptoms suggestive of hypoglycemia occur frequently when patients who have poorly controlled diabetes experience improved glycemic control. These symptoms of pseudohypoglycemia occur at blood glucose levels that are usually within the physiologic range or even higher, and are attributable to altered glycemic threshold for release of counterregulatory hormones [71]. Patients undergoing intensification of diabetes management should be warned of the phenomenon of pseudohypoglycemia; many such patients may have unexpressed fears that the symptoms they feel presage imminent hypoglycemic coma. These symptoms and concerns often lead patients to discontinue or inappropriately modify recommended regimens. No specific treatment other than reassurance is indicated for patients who have such episodes of pseudohypoglycemia. After tight glycemic control has been established, patients who experience recurrent hypoglycemia ($<$ 60 mg/dL) are at risk for development of hypoglycemia-associated autonomic failure [72,73], which leads to a blunting of the autonomic responses to and awareness of symptoms of evolving hypoglycemia. The occurrence of iatrogenic hypoglycemia must be avoided or minimized during optimization of glycemic control.

The most widely used approaches include (1) basal insulin (eg, glargine) at bedtime, with continuation of oral agents; (2) split-mixed regimens that deliver a mixture of regular insulin or analogue (lispro, aspart) and an intermediate-acting insulin (NPH), delivered in two injections 12 hours apart; or (3) basal-bolus regimens consisting of basal insulin and premeal boluses of short-acting insulin. Combination regimens of exogenous insulin with sulfonylurea, metformin, TZDs, and α-glucosidase inhibitors are in widespread use. Oftentimes, the insulin requirement can be significantly reduced by concurrent use of a TZD or metformin. The use of sulfonylurea, metformin, or TZD plus bedtime basal insulin is an efficacious strategy for lowering glucose levels, but it must be noted that the sulfonylurea-plus-insulin regimen has no impact on the underlying insulin resistance in type 2 diabetes.

Basal insulin can be started as bedtime NPH or glargine at a low initial dose ($\sim$10 U) and increased by about 4 U every 2 to 3 days (while continuing oral agents) until a fasting blood glucose level of 80 to 120 mg/dL is achieved [74]. Obviously, patient cooperation in monitoring and relaying home blood glucose levels to the clinic is critical to the success of this titration approach. In the Treat-to-Target trial [74], the average bedtime dose of basal insulin (NPH or glargine) needed to achieve a fasting plasma glucose level of about 100 mg/dL was approximately 50 U. Patients who do not achieve a fasting glucose target of 80 to 120 mg/dL despite injecting more than 50 U of basal insulin at bedtime may require multiple injections of mixed short- and longer-acting insulin preparations for optimal control. Typically, large daily doses of insulin ($>$ 100 U/d) are required to maintain optimal glycemic control in patients who have type 2 diabetes, although concurrent use of insulin-sensitizer drugs may decrease insulin requirement.

The notable side effects of insulin therapy include weight gain and hypoglycemia, the latter being infrequent in patients who have type 2 diabetes. There is no evidence that insulin therapy increases cardiovascular risk in patients who have diabetes. Indeed, in the UKPDS there was a 16% reduction in myocardial infarction in the group treated with insulin or sulfonylurea, compared with the diet-treated control group [26].

Barriers to effective diabetes care

Despite the plethora of effective therapeutic options for the treatment of diabetes, evidence indicates that glycemic control falls short of national guidelines [35]. Suboptimal treatment of diabetes in ethnic minorities can be attributed to barriers at the patient, provider, and health systems levels.

Patient-level barriers

These include poor diabetes-specific knowledge; negative belief and attitudes about diabetes; lack of self-management skills; and nonadherence to lifestyle behaviors that improve diabetes control, such as physical activity and diet [75–78]. Other barriers include mismatch of patient and physician expectations in diabetes self-management, differential socioeconomic levels that impede physician-patient communication, and distrust of physician recommendations by ethnic minority patients that may decrease adherence [79,80]. Language barriers and low literacy rates among ethnic minority patients who have diabetes also impede physician-patient communication [80,81].

Other important patient-level barriers to the inculcation of diabetes self-management skills include lack of a locus of control [82] and fatalism [83]. Locus of control in the context of diabetes care refers to the person or source that patients often identify as holding the key to their health [84]. For most chronic metabolic disorders that require the implementation of multiple self-care tasks (eg, diet, exercise, glucose monitoring, taking medications per schedule, and so forth), the proper locus of control should be internal (ie, centered within the patient). Externality in locus of control predicts negative outcomes [84]. Patients who correctly accept responsibility and take control do better than those who externalize the locus of control. A major goal of the doctor-patient encounter in diabetes should be to assist patients in moving from an external to an internal locus of control.

Fatalism is another potential patient-level barrier. Fatalism is defined as "a doctrine that events are fixed in advance so that human beings are powerless to change them" [85]. In a recent qualitative study [83], fatalism was found to be associated with diabetes self-management in African Americans who have type 2 diabetes. Fatalism was found to characterize the nature of the interaction between the individual who has diabetes and others, the meanings they attached to such interactions, and the decision to adopt an effective or ineffective diabetes self-management behavior [83]. Fatalistic patients were less likely to adopt effective diabetes self-management behavior. Health providers may need to explore the role of fatalistic beliefs as a barrier to adoption of effective lifestyle changes in African Americans who have type 2 diabetes.

Provider and system barriers

Provider-level barriers include negative beliefs and attitudes about diabetes [86], perceived complexity and difficulty of treating diabetes [87,88], lack of adequate time and resources for diabetes treatment [88,89], and clinical inertia [90–92]. Health systems barriers include accessibility, availability and convenience of appointments, organization of care, availability of interpreters, health insurance coverage, reimbursement levels, and formulary restrictions.

Summary and future directions

To achieve sustained improvements in overall quality of care for diabetes and to reduce the disproportionate burden of disease in ethnic minorities, critical changes in the current delivery of care to individuals who have diabetes are needed. The necessary changes include a shift from an acute model of care to a chronic disease care model, adoption of patient-centered and collaborative management approaches, and increased health provider and health systems accountability for quality diabetes care.

Chronic disease model of care

The chronic disease model [93,94] needs to become the standard for clinical management of diabetes. The chronic care model identifies the essential elements of a system that encourages high-quality chronic disease management. The major components of the model include the community, the health system, self-management support, delivery system design, decision support, and clinical information systems [95]. There is increasing evidence that the chronic disease model improves clinical outcomes for diabetes [96–99]. Health care systems and clinical practices need to recognize the benefit of creating effective practice teams, incorporating evidence-based clinical practice guidelines in day-to-day clinical care, and using clinical information systems to provide reminder and feedback to health care providers. Health care providers need to encourage greater patient autonomy, increase patient and family involvement in clinical decision-making, and increase use of ancillary services and community resources to improve patient outcomes.

Patient-centered and collaborative care approaches

Patient-centered care acknowledges that patients are primarily responsible for day-to-day diabetes management. The main objective is to empower patients to manage their disease better. Collaborative management is said to have occurred when patients and providers have shared goals and there is clear delineation of roles and responsibilities between patients and health providers [100]. This requires mutual understanding and respect of the different roles and responsibilities. The most benefit from collaborative management is achieved when trust, goal sharing, and motivation are instilled by physicians [101–103]. It entails equipping patients with necessary diabetes self-management skills to improve outcomes [104–109]. As patients become more educated about their chronic illness, there are more requests for self-management support. This is likely to result in increased use of the services of diabetes educators, nutritionists, dietitians, social workers, psychologists, and pharmacists with the goal of achieving optimal diabetes control and improved health outcomes.

Health systems accountability

There is a need to hold health care providers and health systems accountable for the quality of diabetes care provided. Quality improvement efforts by the American Diabetes Association and the Centers for Medicare and Medicaid Services need to be tied into reimbursement. Strategies need to be developed to identify and reward health providers and health systems that provide optimal diabetes care. Similarly, there is a need to implement disincentives to providers and systems that provide suboptimal diabetes care based on acceptable national standards.

Primary prevention of type 2 diabetes

Once diabetes has developed, it is incurable and expensive to manage. As the leading cause of end-stage renal failure, blindness, amputation, and heart disease, the case for primary prevention of diabetes is compelling and self-evident. The grim economic, sociocultural, and clinical disparities have already been discussed in the context of ethnic minorities in diabetes. Under the scenario of an escalating epidemic of type 2 diabetes and its complications, a stronger case cannot be made for an aggressive focus on primary prevention as a top national priority, especially among disadvantaged populations.

In the Diabetes Prevention Program [18], lifestyle modification or metformin therapy significantly reduced the risk of development of type 2 diabetes in persons who have impaired glucose tolerance from African-, Hispanic-, Asian-, Native-, and European-American ethnic backgrounds. Subjects from all ethnic extractions responded equally, and there was no evidence of ethnic disparities in the effectiveness of the interventions used to prevent diabetes in the Diabetes Prevention Program. Nonpharmacologic approaches to the prevention of type 2 diabetes generally prove more efficacious than expensive medications [18,110]. These approaches are the interventions of choice. The translation of diabetes prevention through dietary modification and increased physical activity at the community level is a challenge that all health care providers, policy makers, and health systems administrators ought to embrace with enthusiasm.

References

[1] National Institute of Diabetes and Digestive and Kidney Diseases. National diabetes statistics fact sheet: general information and national estimates on diabetes in the United States. NIH Publication No. 04–3892. Bethesda (MD): US Department of Health and Human Services, National Institutes of Health; 2004.

[2] American Diabetes Association. Diagnosis and classification of diabetes mellitus. Diabetes Care 2005;28:S37–42.

[3] National Institute of Diabetes and Digestive and Kidney Diseases. Diabetes in African Americans. NIH Publication No. 02–3266. Bethesda (MD): US Department of Health and Human Services, National Institutes of Health; 2002.

[4] American Diabetes Association. Screening for type 2 diabetes. Diabetes Care 2004;27: S11–4.

[5] Executive Summary of the Third Report of the National Cholesterol Education Program (NCEP) Expert Panel on Detection, Evaluation, and Treatment of High Blood Cholesterol in Adults (Adult Treatment Panel III). JAMA 2001;285:2486–97.

[6] Neel JV, Weder AB, Julius S. Type II diabetes, essential hypertension, and obesity as "syndromes of impaired genetic homeostasis": the "thrifty genotype" hypothesis enters the 21st century. Perspect Biol Med 1998;42:44–74.

[7] Stunkard AJ. Current views on obesity. Am J Med 1996;100:230–6.

[8] Sobal J, Stunkard A. Socioeconomic status of obesity: a review of the literature. Psychol Bull 1989;105:260–75.

[9] Lev-Ran A. Thrifty genotype: how applicable is it to obesity and type 2 diabetes? Diabetes Rev 1999;7:1–22.

[10] Curtsinger JW, Service P, Prout T. Antagonistic pleiotropy, reversal of dominance, and genetic polymorphism. Am Nat 1994;144:210–28.

[11] Turner RC, Levy JC, Clark A. Complex genetics of type 2 diabetes: thrifty genes and previously neutral polymorphisms. Q J Med 1993;86:413–7.

[12] Knowler WC, Nelson RG, Saad MF, et al. Determinants of diabetes mellitus in the Pima Indians. Diabetes Care 1993;16:216–27.

[13] Serjeantson S, Owerbach D, Zimmet P, et al. Genetics of diabetes in Nauru: effects of foreign admixture, HLA antigens, and the insulin-gene linked polymorphism. Diabetologia 1983;25:13–7.

[14] Groop LC, Tuomi T. Non-insulin-dependent diabetes mellitus: a collision between thrifty genes and affluent society. Ann Med 1997;29:37–53.

[15] Fujimoto W. Diabetes in Asian and Pacific Islander Americans. In: Harris MI, Cowie CC, Stern MP, et al, editors. Diabetes in America. 2nd edition. Bethesda (MD): National Diabetes Data Group, National Institutes of Health; 1995. p. 661–81.

[16] Harris M. Noninsulin-dependent diabetes mellitus in black and white Americans. Diabet Metab Rev 1990;6:71–90.

[17] Stern MP, Gaskill SP, Hazuda HP, et al. Does obesity explain excess prevalence of diabetes among Mexican Americans? Result of the San Antonio Heart Study. Diabetologia 1983;24: 272–7.

[18] Diabetes Prevention Program Research Group. Reduction in the incidence of type 2 diabetes with lifestyle intervention or metformin. N Engl J Med 2002;346:393–403.

[19] Goldstein BJ. Insulin resistance as the core defect in type 2 diabetes mellitus. Am J Cardiol 2002;90:3G–10G.

[20] Weyer C, Tataranni PA, Bogardus C, et al. Insulin resistance and insulin secretory dysfunction are independent predictors of worsening of glucose tolerance during each stage of type 2 diabetes development. Diabetes Care 2000;24:89–94.

[21] Osei K, Schuster DP, Owusu SK, et al. Race and ethnicity determine serum insulin and C-peptide concentrations and hepatic insulin extraction and insulin clearance: comparative

studies of three populations of West African ancestry and white Americans. Metabolism 1997;46:53–8.

[22] Osei K, Gaillard T, Schuster DP. Pathogenetic mechanisms of impaired glucose tolerance and type II diabetes in African-Americans. Diabetes Care 1997;20:396–404.

[23] Haffner SM, D'Agostino R, Saad MF, et al. Increased insulin resistance and insulin secretion in nondiabetic African-Americans and Hispanics compared with non-Hispanic whites. Diabetes 1996;45:742–8.

[24] Cowie CC, Harris MI. Physical and metabolic characteristics of persons with diabetes. In: Harris MI, Cowie CC, Stern MP, et al, editors. Diabetes in America. 2nd edition. Bethesda (MD): National Diabetes Data Group, National Institutes of Health; 1995. p. 117–64.

[25] The Diabetes Control and Complications Trial Research Group. The effect of intensive treatment of diabetes on the development and progression of long-term complications in insulin-dependent diabetes mellitus. N Engl J Med 1993;329:978–86.

[26] UK Prospective Diabetes Study Group. Intensive blood-glucose control with sulfonylurea or insulin compared with conventional treatment and risk of complications in patients with type 2 diabetes (UKPDS 33). Lancet 1998;352:837–53.

[27] Harris MI, Klein R, Cowie CC, et al. Is the risk of diabetic retinopathy greater in non-Hispanic blacks and Mexican Americans than in non-Hispanic whites with type 2 diabetes? A US population study. Diabetes Care 1998;21:1230–5.

[28] Martin TI, Selby JV, Zhang D. Physician and patient preventive practices in NIDDM in a large urban managed-care organization. Diabetes Care 1995;18:1124–32.

[29] Egede LE. Lifestyle modification to improve blood pressure control in individuals with diabetes: is physician advice effective? Diabetes Care 2003;26:602–7.

[30] Tull ES, Roseman JM. Diabetes in African Americans. In: Diabetes in America. 2nd edition. Bethesda (MD): National Diabetes Data Group, National Institutes of Health; 1995. p. 613–29.

[31] Wisdom K, Fryzek JP, Havstad SL, et al. Comparison of laboratory test frequency and test results between African-Americans and caucasians with diabetes: opportunity for improvement. Diabetes Care 1997;20:971.

[32] Harris MI. Racial and ethnic differences in health care access and health outcomes for adults with type 2 diabetes. Diabetes Care 2001;24:454–9.

[33] Musey VC, Lee JK, Crawford R, et al. Diabetes in urban African-Americans. 1. Cessation of insulin therapy is the major precipitating cause of diabetic ketoacidosis. Diabetes Care 1995;18:483–9.

[34] Karter AJ, Ferrara A, Liu JY, et al. Ethnic disparities in diabetic complications in an insured population. JAMA 2002;287:2519–27.

[35] Saaddine JB, Engelgau MM, Beckles GL, et al. A diabetes report card for the United States: quality of care in the 1990s. Ann Intern Med 2002;136:565–74.

[36] Egede LE, Zheng D. Racial/ethnic differences in adult vaccination among individuals with diabetes. Am J Public Health 2003;93:324–9.

[37] Egede LE, Zheng D. Racial/ethnic differences in influenza vaccination coverage in high-risk adults. Am J Public Health 2003;93:2074–8.

[38] Egede LE. Association between number of physician visits and influenza vaccination coverage among diabetic adults with access to care. Diabetes Care 2003;26:2562–7.

[39] Cowie CC, Harris MI. Ambulatory medical care for non-Hispanic whites, African-Americans, and Mexican-Americans with NIDDM in the US. Diabetes Care 1997;20:142–7.

[40] Peters AL, Legorreta AP, Ossorio RC, et al. Quality of outpatient care provided to diabetic patients. Diabetes Care 1996;10:601–6.

[41] Jencks SF, Guerdon T, Burwen DR, et al. Quality of medical care delivered to Medicare beneficiaries: a profile at state and national levels. JAMA 2000;284:1670–6.

[42] Huse DM, Oster G, Killen AR, et al. The economic costs of non-insulin-dependent diabetes mellitus. JAMA 1989;262:2708–13.

[43] Druss BG, Marcus SC, Olfson M, et al. Comparing the national economic burden of five chronic conditions. Health Aff (Millwood) 2001;20:233–41.

[44] American Diabetes Association. Economic consequences of diabetes mellitus in the US in 1997. Diabetes Care 1998;21:296–309.

[45] American Diabetes Association. Economic costs of diabetes in the US in 2002. Diabetes Care 2003;26:917–32.

[46] United Kingdom Prospective Diabetes Study Group. UK Prospective Diabetes Study (UKPDS). VIII. Study design, progress and performance. Diabetologia 1991;34: 877–90.

[47] Gray A, Raikou M, McGuire A, et al. Cost effectiveness of an intensive blood glucose control policy in patients with type 2 diabetes: economic analysis alongside randomised controlled trial (UKPDS 41). United Kingdom Prospective Diabetes Study Group. BMJ 2000;320:1373–8.

[48] The CDC Diabetes Cost-effectiveness Group. Cost-effectiveness of intensive glycemic control, intensified hypertension control, and serum cholesterol level reduction for type 2 diabetes. JAMA 2002;287:2542–51.

[49] American Diabetes Association. Standards of medical care for patients with diabetes mellitus. Diabetes Care 2005;28:S4–36.

[50] American Association of Clinical Endocrinologists and the American College of Endocrinology. The American Association of Clinical Endocrinologists medical guidelines for the management of diabetes mellitus: the AACE system of intensive diabetes self-management–2002 update. Endocr Pract 2002;8(Suppl 1):40–82.

[51] Blonde L, Ginsberg BH, Horn S, et al. Frequency of blood glucose monitoring in relation to glycemic control in patients with type 2 diabetes. Diabetes Care 2002;25:245–6.

[52] Ziemer DC, Goldschmid MG, Musey VC, et al. Diabetes in urban African Americans. III. Management of type II diabetes in a municipal hospital setting. Am J Med 1996; 101:25–33.

[53] Grundy SM. Dietary therapy in diabetes mellitus: is there a single best diet? Diabetes Care 1991;14:796–801.

[54] Dagogo-Jack S, Santiago JV. Pathophysiology of type 2 diabetes and modes of action of therapeutic interventions. Arch Intern Med 1997;157:1802–17.

[55] Dagogo-Jack S. Diabetes mellitus and related disorders. In: Ahya S, Flood K, Paranjothi S, editors. Washington manual of medical therapeutics. 30th edition. New York: Lippincott; 2001. p. 455–72.

[56] Moneva M, Dagogo-Jack S. Multiple drug targets in the management of type 2 diabetes mellitus. Curr Drug Targets 2002;3:203–21.

[57] Inzucchi SE, Maggs DG, Spollett GR, et al. Efficacy and metabolic effects of metformin and troglitazone in type 2 diabetes mellitus. N Engl J Med 1998;338:867–72.

[58] Rosen ED, Spiegelman BM. Peroxisome proliferator-activated receptor ligands and atherosclerosis: ending the heartache. J Clin Invest 2000;106:629–31.

[59] Cavaghan MK, Eurmann DA, Byrne MM, et al. Treatment with oral antidiabetic agent troglitazone improves beta cell responses to glucose in subjects with improved glucose tolerance. J Clin Invest 1997;100:530–7.

[60] Osei K, Miller EE, Everitt DE, et al. Rosiglitazone is effective and well tolerated as monotherapy in African Americans with type 2 diabetes. Diabetes 2001;50(Suppl 2):A127.

[61] Liebovitz HE, Dole JF, Patwardhan R, et al. Rosiglitazone monotherapy is effective in patients with type 2 diabetes. J Clin Endocrinol Metab 2001;86:280–8.

[62] Xixing Z, Changyu P, Guangwei L, et al. Rosiglitazone improves glycemic control in Chinese patients with type 2 diabetes mellitus in combination with sulfonylurea. Diabetes 2001;50(Suppl 2):A135.

[63] Gomez-Perez FJ, Fanghanel-Salmon G, Antonio Barbosa J, et al. Efficacy and safety of rosiglitazone plus metformin in Mexicans with type 2 diabetes. Diabetes Metab Res Rev 2002;18:127–34.

[64] Nesto RW, Bell D, Bonow RO, et al. Thiazolidinedione use, fluid retention, and congestive heart failure: a consensus statement from the American Heart Association and American Diabetes Association. Diabetes Care 2004;27:256–63.

[65] Turner RC, Cull CA, Frighi V, et al. Glycemic control with diet, sulfonylurea, metformin, or insulin in patients with type 2 diabetes mellitus: progressive requirement for multiple therapies (UKPDS 49). JAMA 1999;281:2005–12.

[66] Lowe LP, Liu K, Greenland P, et al. Diabetes, asymptomatic hyperglycemia, and 22-year mortality in black and white men. Diabetes Care 1997;20:163–72.

[67] Wolffenbuttel BHR, Gomis R, Squatrito S, et al. Addition of low-dose rosiglitazone to sulphonylurea therapy improves glycaemic control in type 2 diabetic patients. Diabet Med 2000;17:40–7.

[68] Fonseca V, Rosenstock J, Patwardhan R, et al. Effect of metformin and rosiglitazone combination therapy in patients with type 2 diabetes mellitus: a randomized controlled trial. JAMA 2000;283:1695–702.

[69] Jones TA, Sautter M, Van Gaal LF, et al. Addition of rosiglitazone to metformin is most effective in obese, insulin-resistant patients with type 2 diabetes. Diabet Obes Metab 2003;5: 163–70.

[70] UK Prospective Diabetes Study Group. UK Prospective Diabetes Study 16. Overview of 6 years' therapy of type II diabetes: a progressive disease. Diabetes 1995;44:1249–58.

[71] Boyle PJ, Schwartz NS, Shah SD, et al. Plasma glucose concentrations at the onset of hypoglycemic symptoms in patients with poorly controlled diabetes and in nondiabetics. N Engl J Med 1988;318:1487–92.

[72] Dagogo-Jack SE, Craft S, Cryer PE. Hypoglycemia-associated autonomic failure in insulin-dependent diabetes mellitus. J Clin Invest 1993;91:819–28.

[73] Dagogo-Jack S. Hypoglycemia in type 1 diabetes: pathophysiology and prevention. Treat Endocrinol 2004;3:91–103.

[74] Riddle MC, Rosenstock J, Gerich J. The treat-to-target trial: randomized addition of glargine or human NPH insulin to oral therapy of type 2 diabetic patients. Diabetes Care 2003;26:3080–6.

[75] Anderson RM, Herman WH, Davis JM, et al. Barriers to improving diabetes care for blacks [editorial]. Diabetes Care 1991;14:605–9.

[76] Harris MI, Cowie CC, Howie LJ. Self-monitoring of blood glucose by adults with diabetes in the United States population. Diabetes Care 1993;16:1116–23.

[77] Harris MI, Eastman RC, Cowie CC, et al. Racial and ethnic differences in glycemic control of adults with type 2 diabetes. Diabetes Care 1999;22:403–8.

[78] Egede LE, Poston ME. Racial/ethnic differences in leisure-time physical activity levels among individuals with diabetes. Diabetes Care 2004;27:2493–4.

[79] Corbie-Smith G, Thomas SB, Williams MV, et al. Attitudes and beliefs of African Americans toward participation in medical research. J Gen Intern Med 1999;14:537–46.

[80] Schoenberg NE, Amey CH, Coward RT. Diabetes knowledge and sources of information among African American and white older women. Diabetes Educ 1998;24:319–24.

[81] Nurss JR, el-Kebbi IM, Gallina DL, et al. Diabetes in urban African Americans: functional health literacy of municipal hospital outpatients with diabetes. Diabetes Educ 1997;23: 563–8.

[82] Jack L Jr, Airhihenbuwa CO, Namageyo-Funa A, et al. The psychological aspects of diabetes care: using collaborative care to manage older adults with diabetes. Geriatrics 2004;59:26–31.

[83] Egede LE, Bonadonna RJ. Diabetes self-management in African Americans: an exploration of the role of fatalism. Diabetes Educ 2003;29:105–15.

[84] Twenge JM, Zhang L, Im C. It's beyond my control: a cross-temporal meta-analysis of increasing externality in locus of control, 1960–2002. Pers Soc Psychol Rev 2004;8:308–19.

[85] Merriam-Webster's collegiate dictionary. 10th edition. Springfield (MA): Merriam-Webster; 1998.

[86] Egede LE, Michel Y. Attitudes of internal medicine physicians toward type 2 diabetes. South Med J 2002;95:88–91.

[87] Larme AC, Pugh JA. Attitudes of primary care providers toward diabetes: barriers to guideline implementation. Diabetes Care 1998;21:1391–6.

[88] Egede LE, Michel Y. Perceived difficulty of diabetes treatment in primary care: does it differ by patient ethnicity? Diabetes Educ 2001;27:678–84.

[89] Barnes CS, Ziemer DC, Miller CD, et al. Little time for diabetes management in the primary care setting. Diabetes Educ 2004;30:126–35.

[90] el-Kebbi IM, Ziemer DC, Musey VC, et al. Diabetes in urban African-Americans. IX. Provider adherence to management protocols. Diabetes Care 1997;20:698–703.

[91] Cook CB, Ziemer DC, El-Kebbi IM, et al. Diabetes in urban African-Americans. XVI. Overcoming clinical inertia improves glycemic control in patients with type 2 diabetes. Diab Care 1999;22(9):1494–500.

[92] Phillips LS, Branch WT, Cook CB, et al. Clinical inertia. Ann Intern Med 2001;135:825–34.

[93] Wagner EH. Population-based management of diabetes care. Patient Educ Couns 1995;26:225–30.

[94] Wagner EH, Austin BT, Von Korff M. Organizing care for patients with chronic illness. Milbank Q 1996;74:511–44.

[95] Bodenheimer T, Wagner EH, Grumbach K. Improving primary care for patients with chronic illness. JAMA 2002;288:1775–9.

[96] Wagner EH, Glasgow RE, Davis C, et al. Quality improvement in chronic illness care: a collaborative approach. Jt Comm J Qual Improv 2001;27:63–80.

[97] Wagner EH, Grothaus LC, Sandhu N, et al. Chronic care clinics for diabetes in primary care: a system-wide randomized trial. Diabetes Care 2001;24:695–700.

[98] Bodenheimer T, Wagner EH, Grumbach K. Improving primary care for patients with chronic illness: the chronic care model, Part 2. JAMA 2002;288:1909–14.

[99] Glasgow RE, Funnell MM, Bonomi AE, et al. Self-management aspects of the improving chronic illness care breakthrough series: implementation with diabetes and heart failure teams. Ann Behav Med 2002;24:80–7.

[100] Von Korff M, Gruman J, Schaefer J, et al. Collaborative management of chronic illness. Ann Intern Med 1997;127:1097–102.

[101] Toobert DJ, Glasgow RE. Problem solving and diabetes self-care. J Behav Med 1991;14:71–86.

[102] Clement S. Diabetes self-management education. Diabetes Care 1995;18:1204–14.

[103] Glasgow RE, Wagner EH, Kaplan RM, et al. If diabetes is a public health problem, why not treat it as one? A population-based approach to chronic illness. Ann Behav Med 1999;21:159–70.

[104] McCaul KD, Glasgow RE, Schafer LC. Diabetes regimen behaviors: predicting adherence. Med Care 1987;25:868–81.

[105] Glasgow RE. A practical model of diabetes management and education. Diabetes Care 1995;18:117–26.

[106] Anderson RM, Funnell MM, Barr PA, et al. Learning to empower patients: results of professional education program for diabetes educators. Diabetes Care 1991;14:584–90.

[107] Anderson RM, Fitzgerald JT, Funnell MM, et al. Evaluation of an activated patient diabetes education newsletter. Diabetes Educ 1994;20:29–34.

[108] Anderson RM, Funnell MM, Butler PM, et al. Patient empowerment: results of a randomized controlled trial. Diabetes Care 1995;18:943–9.

[109] Ruggiero L, Glasgow R, Dryfoos JM, et al. Diabetes self-management: self-reported recommendations and patterns in a large population. Diabetes Care 1997;20:568–76.

[110] Tuomilehto J, Lindstrom J, Eriksson JG, et al. Finnish Diabetes Prevention Study Group. Prevention of type 2 diabetes mellitus by changes in lifestyle among subjects with impaired glucose tolerance. N Engl J Med 2001;344:1343–50.

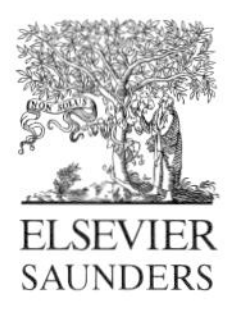
ELSEVIER
SAUNDERS

Med Clin N Am 89 (2005) 977–1001

THE MEDICAL
CLINICS
OF NORTH AMERICA

Issues in Minority Health: Atherosclerosis and Coronary Heart Disease in African Americans

Luther T. Clark, MD

Division of Cardiovascular Medicine, Department of Medicine, State University of New York Downstate Medical Center, 450 Clarkson Avenue, Box 1199, Brooklyn, New York 11203, USA

Cardiovascular disease, and in particular, coronary heart disease (CHD) is the leading cause of death in the United States for Americans of both sexes and of all racial and ethnic backgrounds [1–5]. African Americans have the highest overall CHD mortality rate and the highest out-of-hospital coronary death rate of any ethnic group in the United States, particularly at younger ages (Box 1) [6–10]. In addition, compared with whites, African Americans have a higher annual rate of first myocardial infarction at all ages (Fig. 1) [1].

The reasons for the earlier onset of CHD and excess CHD deaths among African Americans have not been fully elucidated; however, it is evident that a high prevalence of coronary risk factors, patient delays in seeking medical care, delays in diagnosis and treatment of high-risk individuals, and limited access to cardiovascular care (preventive, maintenance, and procedures such as cardiac catheterization, coronary interventions, and bypass surgery) are important contributors.

The clinical spectrum of acute and chronic CHD in African Americans is the same as in whites; however, the higher rate of out-of-hospital sudden cardiac death and an apparent propensity for catastrophic events during myocardial ischemia has led to the hypothesis of a more susceptible underlying anatomic substrate in African Americans who have CHD that may increase predisposition to malignant arrhythmias and sudden death during ischemia [11].

In this review, the magnitude of the burden of CHD in African Americans, the biologic factors contributing to excess risk, and opportunities for

E-mail address: ltclark@downstate.edu

Box 1. Coronary heart disease in African Americans compared with whites

Earlier age of onset of CHD
Higher overall mortality from CHD
Higher out-of-hospital mortality
Higher sudden cardiac death rate
Higher annual rate of first myocardial infarction at all ages

---

developing more effective prevention and treatment strategies are examined. The terms *African American* and *black* are used synonymously and interchangeably.

Historical perspective

Disparities in outcomes from various diseases between blacks and whites have been documented for as long as records have been kept. More than a century ago, when the National Medical Association was founded in 1895 as the voice of black physicians and the patients they serve, one of the key objectives of the group was improving the health status and outcomes of African Americans and the disadvantaged [12]. Clinical studies comparing cardiovascular disease prevalence and outcomes in blacks and whites date at

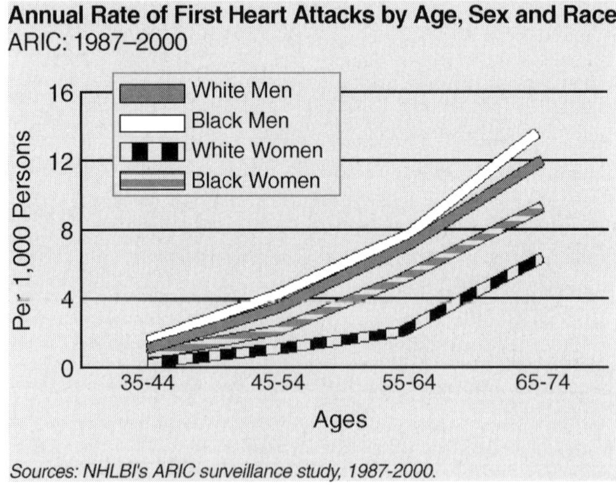

Fig. 1. Annual rate of first heart attacks by age, sex, and race. (*From* American Heart Association. Annual rate of first heart attacks by age, sex, and race, ARIC: 1987–2000. National Heart, Lung, and Blood Institute Atherosclerosis Risk in Communities surveillance study. Heart disease and stroke statistics—2005 update. Available at: http://www.americanheart.org. Accessed March 14, 2005; with permission.)

least as far back as the 1920s when Stone and Vanzant [13] reported that hypertensive heart disease was twice as frequent in blacks as in whites but that arteriosclerotic heart disease and angina pectoris were uncommon in blacks. It is interesting to note that even in the 1920s, some prominent clinicians believed that cardiac ischemia and angina occurred similarly in blacks and whites but was often missed in blacks because of misinterpretation of symptoms (ie, the propensity of some blacks to describe their symptoms as "misery in the stomach" or "misery in the chest") [13], expressions that are sometimes still used today. Thus, although hypertension and hypertensive heart disease were recognized as important causes of cardiovascular disease in blacks during the early twentieth century, coronary artery disease was not recognized as an important problem until decades later.

One of the most comprehensive analyses of the disparity in the burden of death and illness from cardiovascular diseases experienced by African Americans and other minorities relative to the population as a whole appeared in 1985 when the Task Force on Black and Minority Health, convened by the secretary of the Department of Health and Human Services, released its report on black and minority health [14]. This report (released August 1985) provided a comprehensive analysis of the scope and magnitude of cardiovascular and cerebrovascular diseases in blacks and other minorities. One of the major findings was that among blacks, there was an excess of approximately 60,000 (preventable) deaths annually, most of which were due to cardiovascular diseases. In 2002, the Institute of Medicine added to the growing body of literature documenting the continuing existence of health disparities in America with its report, *Unequal Treatment: Confronting Racial and Ethnic Disparities in Health Care* [15]. This report further underscored the need to address disparities in the burden of death and illness experienced by African Americans relative to the population as a whole. Focusing on the issue of treatment, the Institute of Medicine report concluded that racial and ethnic minorities receive lower quality health care than whites, even when they are insured to the same degree and when other health care access–related factors such as the ability to pay for care are the same. Further documentation of the strength of the evidence for disparities in cardiovascular care was provided in the Henry J. Kaiser Family Foundation's 2002 report, *Racial/Ethnic Differences in Cardiac Care: the Weight of the Evidence* [16]. In an analysis of 81 studies addressing racial/ethnic differences in cardiac care, this report added to previous analyses and affirmed that (1) African Americans are less likely than whites to receive appropriate and necessary treatments for cardiac disease, including thrombolytics, catheterization, angioplasty, and bypass surgery; and (2) these racial/ethnic differences in care remain after adjustment for clinical and socioeconomic factors.

These landmark reports further documented and heightened awareness of a continuing national paradox in the United States: although there has been tremendous scientific achievements in terms of improvement in overall health status for the general population, significant health inequities persist among African Americans and other minorities.

Coronary risk factors

African Americans have an excess burden of major risk factors for coronary artery disease [1,4,5,7,17–19] and are more likely to have multiple risk factors than whites [17–19]. The predictive value of most conventional risk factors appears to be similar in African Americans and whites [20]; however, the risk of death and other sequelae attributable to some risk factors (eg, hypertension and diabetes) is greater [21–23] and the risk of certain others such as lipoprotein(a) [Lp(a)] is lower for African Americans [24–27]. Hypertension, left ventricular hypertrophy, type 2 diabetes mellitus, obesity, cigarette smoking, and physical inactivity occur more frequently in African Americans (Box 2). Because these risk factors are modifiable, there is great opportunity for prevention; however, the combination of lower screening and less effective treatment of risk factors contributes to worse outcomes and health disparities. Directed public education campaigns about cardiac risk factors and their contributions to cardiovascular disease and disparities and about the importance of risk factor modification is important for improving outcomes and eliminating cardiovascular disparities.

Hypertension

Systolic hypertension and diastolic hypertension are established risk factors for cardiovascular disease. Systolic blood pressure is a better

---

Box 2. Coronary heart disease risk factors more prevalent in African Americans compared with whites

Associated with increased coronary heart disease risk
  Hypertension
  Type 2 diabetes mellitus
  Obesity
  Cigarette smoking
  Physical inactivity
  Left ventricular hypertrophy

Association with coronary heart disease risk unclear
  Higher Lp(a)

Associated with decreased coronary heart disease risk?
  Higher high-density lipoprotein cholesterol

predictor than diastolic blood pressure of risk for CHD, heart failure, stroke, end-stage renal disease, and overall mortality. In African Americans, hypertension is more prevalent, develops at a younger age, and is associated with a three to five times higher cardiovascular mortality rate than in whites [20–22,28–30]. African Americans also appear to experience greater cardiovascular and renal damage at any level of blood pressure than whites, although the higher mortality rates in hypertensive African Americans may reflect greater disease severity and more left ventricular hypertrophy [20–22].

In addition to recommendations in the *Seventh Report of the Joint National Committee on Prevention, Detection, Evaluation, and Treatment of High Blood Pressure* [31], a consensus statement on the management of hypertension in African Americans was recently published by the International Society on Hypertension in Blacks [32] that provided a practical, evidence-based clinical tool for achieving blood pressure goals. All adults should know their blood pressure and whether it is elevated. If elevated, patients should obtain treatment and know what the treated blood pressure goal is. Lifestyle modifications that have been shown to lower blood pressure (weight loss, aerobic exercise, reductions in dietary sodium and saturated fat intake, and increased intake of dietary potassium) should be emphasized. The benefits of lifestyle modifications include the ability to attain goal blood pressure levels with fewer antihypertensive medications and with favorable effects on other cardiovascular risk factors.

Diabetes mellitus

Diabetes mellitus increases risk for CHD at least twofold to fourfold [33–34]. Furthermore, vascular complications in patients who have diabetes appear at a younger age, affect women as often as men, and are more often fatal than in patients who do not have diabetes [33–37]. Atherosclerotic plaques in patients who have diabetes appear to be morphologically similar to those in patients who do not have diabetes and differ only by the extent and severity of atherosclerotic disease. African Americans and other nonwhite minorities have a greater burden of diabetes, and its vascular complications are greater than in whites [23,38,39]. The prevalence of type 2 diabetes mellitus in African Americans is two to three times higher than in whites [23,36,38,39]. In the United States, approximately 11.4% (2.7 million) of African Americans aged 20 years or older have diabetes.

Risk factor clustering and the metabolic syndrome

African Americans are more likely than whites to have multiple CHD risk factors [17–19]. The presence of multiple risk factors increases CHD risk synergistically. Although the etiology of risk factor clustering is unknown, genetic and environmental factors have been implicated. The metabolic syndrome—also known as insulin resistance syndrome, metabolic syndrome X, and dysmetabolic syndrome—refers to a specific clustering of cardiovascular risk factors in the same individual (abdominal obesity, atherogenic dyslipidemia, elevated blood pressure, insulin resistance, a prothrombotic state, and a proinflammatory state) (Table 1) [40]. Patients who have the metabolic syndrome are at increased risk for the development of diabetes and cardiovascular disease. According to a recent analysis of data from the Third National Health and Nutritional Examination Survey (NHANES III), approximately 47 million Americans (23.7% of the population) have the metabolic syndrome [41]. African-American women and Hispanic men and women have the highest prevalences of the metabolic syndrome [42,43], which may be attributable to the disproportionate occurrence of elevated blood pressure, obesity, and diabetes in African Americans and the high prevalence of obesity in Hispanics. Management of the metabolic syndrome consists primarily of modification or reversal of its root causes and direct therapy of the risk factors. The first strategy involves weight reduction and increased physical activity, both of which can improve all components of the syndrome. The second strategy involves treatment of the individual risk factors to further improve blood pressure, lipids, and glucose, thereby decreasing the risk of cardiovascular disease. According to one recent analysis [43], aggressive management of elevated blood pressure and dyslipidemia in individuals with the metabolic syndrome and control to optimal levels could result in the prevention of more than 80% of cardiovascular events.

Obesity

Obesity increases risk for CHD, stroke, hypertension, and type 2 diabetes mellitus in adults and is a major component of the metabolic syndrome [44,45]. The abdominal pattern of obesity (specifically, visceral adiposity)

Table 1
Clinical identification of the metabolic syndrome

Risk factor	Defining level
Abdominal obesity (waist circumference)	
Men	>102 cm (>40 in)
Women	>88 cm (>35 in)
Triglycerides	
HDL cholesterol	
Men	<40 mg/dL
Women	<50 mg/dL
Blood pressure	≥130/85 mm Hg
Fasting glucose	≥110 mg/dL

From Third Report of the National Cholesterol Education Program (NCEP) Expert Panel on Detection, Evaluation, and Treatment of High Blood Cholesterol in Adults (Adult Treatment Panel III). Final report. Circulation 2002;106:3143; with permission.

appears to be the most hazardous and atherogenic. The increased risk appears to be mediated chiefly through its metabolic consequences (ie, insulin resistance, glucose intolerance, hypertriglyceridemia, reduced HDL cholesterol, and hypertension). Obesity in the United States population has steadily increased over the past several decades in all educational, sex, age, and ethnic groups [46–48]. During the interval between the Second National Health and Nutritional Examination Survey (1976–1980) and NHANES III (1999–2000), the age-adjusted prevalence of obesity increased from 15.0% to 30.5% [47,48]. In the year 2000, there were 38.8 million adults who were defined as obese, with a body mass index >30 kg/m^2, representing a 61% increase since 1991 [46–48]. This increasing epidemic of obesity and the recent recognition that more than 60% of Americans are overweight or obese underscore the urgency of recognizing and treating the metabolic syndrome and the need for aggressive approaches to weight reduction for these individuals [46]. The prevalence of obesity among African-American men is similar to that among white men. In African-American women, however, obesity is twice as prevalent and the abdominal pattern of obesity is more common than in their white counterparts [46–49].

Dyslipidemia

Total and low-density lipoprotein cholesterol

Approximately 25% of adult African Americans in the general population have high-risk lipid profiles. Elevated total or low-density lipoprotein cholesterol (LDL-C) levels are established independent risk factors for CHD, and reductions in LDL-C have decreased the risk for CHD events in several large clinical outcome trials. Most population-based studies report that African Americans have similar or lower total serum cholesterol levels than whites and a lower prevalence of hypercholesterolemia [5,17–19,50–53]. The relationship between total cholesterol levels and CHD mortality is the same among African Americans as among whites [51].

High-density lipoprotein cholesterol

Low high-density lipoprotein cholesterol (HDL-C) levels increase the risk for development of CHD independent of LDL-C levels and other risk factors, whereas elevated HDL-C levels are protective. The National Cholesterol Education Progam's adult treatment guidelines [40] define low HDL-C as < 40 mg/dL in men and women. For diagnosis of the metabolic syndrome, however, HDL < 40 mg/dL in men or < 50 mg/dL in women is considered abnormal and one of the diagnostic criteria. Low HDL-C is a strong and independent predictor of CHD [40,54]. HDL-C levels are higher in African Americans, particularly in African-American men, than in their white counterparts [40,50–53]. The underlying mechanisms for this physiology have not been fully elucidated but may relate to a genetically lower activity of hepatic lipase [55].

Triglycerides

Elevated serum triglyceride levels (>150 mg/dL) are associated with increased risk for CHD [56]. Causes of hypertriglyceridemia include obesity and overweight status, physical inactivity, a high-carbohydrate diet (>60% of calories), diabetes mellitus, certain drugs (estrogens, corticosteroids), and excessive alcohol intake. Elevated triglyceride levels are associated with low HDL-C levels, small low-density lipoprotein particles, procoagulant effects, hypertension, and insulin resistance—factors that can increase the risk of developing atherosclerosis. Triglyceride levels in African-American men and women are generally lower than in white men and women who have CHD and who do not have CHD [40,50–53].

Lipoprotein(a)

Lp(a) levels are two to three times higher in African Americans than in whites [5,24–27]. Prospective studies evaluating the role of Lp(a) levels as a predictor of cardiovascular events demonstrate conflicting results. Several studies have reported that Lp(a) levels are an independent risk factor for CHD in whites [24–27]; however, the role of Lp(a) levels as a determinant of CHD risk in African Americans remains unknown. Recent trials in African Americans that evaluated the relationship of Lp(a) levels and atherosclerosis failed to detect an association [24–27].

Because the atherogenicity of Lp(a) appears to differ in whites and blacks, it has been hypothesized that this may be due to the presence of a greater predominance of small apolipoprotein A isoforms (associated with CHD) in whites than in blacks [57].

Cigarette smoking

Cigarette smoking is a powerful risk factor for atherosclerosis and CHD. More African-American men smoke than white men, but African-American men consume fewer cigarettes per day [1,58]. African-American and white women smoke at comparable rates [1,58]. Despite smoking fewer cigarettes per day, African Americans have lower cessation rates and experience higher rates of smoking-related health complications. Because of the high preference for menthol cigarettes among African-American smokers, it has been hypothesized that smoking menthol cigarettes may contribute to the excess smoking-related morbidity and the less successful smoking cessation rates among African Americans [59].

Physical inactivity

Physical inactivity is associated with increased risk for CHD, whereas physical activity favorably modifies CHD risk [60,61]. Physical inactivity reduces caloric expenditure, contributes to obesity and other CHD risk factors, and adversely affects cardiovascular fitness and function. Physical activity decreases cardiovascular risk and favorably affects a number of

CHD risk factors including elevated blood pressure, insulin resistance, dyslipidemia, obesity, and the metabolic syndrome. African Americans have a higher prevalence of physical inactivity and are less likely to get the recommended amounts of exercise than their white counterparts [5,17–19].

Inflammatory markers and other emerging risk factors

Vascular inflammation has recently been recognized as an important contributor to the etiology, progression, and complications of atherosclerosis [62,63]. Elevated inflammatory markers in prospective trials have been associated with increased cardiovascular risk among healthy individuals and those at higher risk because of the presence of other risk factors or known coronary disease. Some but not all standard therapies for prevention of cardiovascular disease have anti-inflammatory effects, effects that might contribute importantly to their observed clinical benefits. Blood-based markers of inflammation include C-reactive protein, fibrinogen, serum albumin, leukocyte count, serum amyloid A, and others [62]. The most extensively studied inflammatory marker is C-reactive protein, an acute-phase protein produced by the liver in response to cytokine production during tissue injury, inflammation, or infection. The potential role of vascular inflammation as a direct target of therapy and the extent to which reducing vascular inflammation is beneficial in terms of cardiovascular disease prevention remain largely speculative and are yet to be determined in clinical trials.

Data on inflammatory biomarkers and their significance for risk assessment and treatment of cardiovascular diseases in African Americans are beginning to emerge but remain limited [63,64]. Some studies have reported higher C-reactive protein levels in African Americans than in whites, but the significance of this finding remains unclear [63,64]. African Americans have also been found to have higher fibrinogen levels and enhanced fibrinolytic activity (and better responses to fibrinolytic therapy) compared with whites.

Coronary heart disease

CHD and its thrombotic complications are major causes of morbidity and mortality in the United States. There are a number of reported differences between blacks and whites as to the extent of underlying atherosclerosis, markers of inflammation, hemostasis, endothelial dysfunction, and coronary vasospasm [5]. Most of the reported differences have been modest and their clinical importance in diagnosing and treating coronary syndromes are not well documented. Nevertheless, there continues to be considerable interest in the differences in the clinical manifestations and underlying pathobiology of CHD in various ethnic groups. Some of the interest has emerged because of an increased appreciation of the significance of CHD in these groups and some because of their apparent inconsistency with generally accepted pathophysiologic concepts. In the case of African Americans, the two most often cited apparent paradoxes are (1) despite the greater burden of certain coronary risk factors in African Americans, the incidence of angiographically significant coronary artery disease is lower in African Americans than in whites [5,65–67]; and (2) despite less severe coronary disease on angiography and fewer Q wave infarctions in African Americans, CHD events occur at younger ages and are associated with higher mortality rates in African Americans than in whites [5,8–10,68]. Although issues of socioeconomic status, access to cardiovascular care, and patients' health care–seeking behaviors contribute to clinical outcomes, recent advances in understanding the pathophysiology of acute coronary events also provide possible insights into biologic similarities and differences.

Pathobiology

Extent of underlying coronary atherosclerosis

Although a number of studies have reported less severe obstructive coronary artery disease on angiography in blacks compared with whites [65–67], some investigators have reported a more extensive burden of atherosclerotic disease among blacks than among their white counterparts [69]. The absence of significant obstructive coronary disease in high-risk patients should not necessarily be interpreted as benign because the biology of atherosclerotic lesions and their instability may be a more important determinant of risk for CHD events than the obstructive severity of lesions. The degree of luminal stenosis does not correlate well with acute myocardial infarction in any other population group and should not be expected to correlate in African Americans. In patients who have significant vasoconstrictive and/or microvascular disease, myocardial ischemia can occur in the absence of significant obstructive epicardial coronary artery disease. It is unknown whether these disorders are more common in African Americans.

Plaque instability, inflammation, and microembolization

Atherosclerosis is present in most adults in the United States; however, acute coronary syndromes (ACSs) and other clinical events occur primarily when an arterial wall becomes inflamed and atherosclerotic plaques fissure, crack, or rupture. Inflammation plays an important role in the etiology, progression, and acute complications of atherosclerosis. Histologically, disrupted atheromatous plaques obtained at autopsy have demonstrated the presence of heavy infiltration of active macrophage foam cells. Culprit lesions responsible for ACSs contain significantly more inflammatory cells than lesions found in patients who have stable angina pectoris. The most common site of plaque rupture is in the shoulder region of the plaque, where inflammatory cells are most prominent. Inflammatory mediators may influence macrophages, endothelial cells, and smooth muscle cells, resulting in plaque weakening and disruption [70–72].

Embolization of platelet aggregates in the microcirculation also plays an important role in the cardiac damage associated with ACSs, and obstruction of the microcirculation can lead to myocardial damage, arrhythmias, and cardiac death. Although there is no evidence that these phenomena occur more often in African Americans than in whites, their importance in ACSs, particularly unstable angina and non–Q wave infarction, appears to be greater than previously appreciated.

Endothelial dysfunction and coronary vasospasm

Endothelial dysfunction plays an important role in the pathogenesis of ischemic heart disease and may be an early manifestation of atherosclerosis [73–76]. In patients who have hypertension and left ventricular hypertrophy, endothelial dysfunction occurs as a maladaptive change even when there is minimal or no angiographic evidence of coronary disease [77–81]. The prognostic significance of endothelial dysfunction in African Americans is unknown. Endothelin-1 is a potent vasoconstrictor peptide secreted by endothelial cells. Plasma endothelin-1 levels are higher in hypertensive African Americans compared with hypertensive whites [81]. Moreover, left ventricular hypertrophy has a greater impact on endothelial dysfunction in African Americans than in whites [79,81].

Underlying anatomic substrate

African Americans have a high prevalence of underlying hypertension and left ventricular hypertrophy that may increase predisposition to lethal arrhythmias and potentially lethal silent ischemic events [11]. Because left ventricular hypertrophy increases risk in all populations in which it has been studied, the increased risk in African Americans is expected. The higher frequency of type 2 diabetes mellitus may also contribute to differences in clinical manifestations and predisposition to ischemic events and arrhythmias.

Acute coronary syndromes

ACSs encompass a spectrum of manifestations of unstable coronary artery disease, including unstable angina, non–ST-segment elevation myocardial infarction, ST-segment elevation myocardial infarction, and sudden cardiac death. Clinical trials investigating ACSs and clinical management guidelines often group together patients who have unstable angina and those who have non–ST-segment elevation myocardial infarction. These two entities have similar manifestations, and a distinction between them can usually be made only after several hours when the results of cardiac enzymes become available.

In the United States, approximately 1.7 million individuals are hospitalized annually with unstable angina and acute myocardial infarction [1]. Coronary atherosclerosis is the most common underlying pathology. Acute cardiac events are usually triggered by plaque rupture, fissuring, erosion with superimposed thrombosis, and coronary vasospasm [70–74]. Clinically, ACSs are heterogeneous disorders with risk of death and recurrent cardiac ischemic events that vary among individuals and population subgroups. The heterogeneity of clinical presentations and outcomes is related to multiple factors, including (1) the extent of underlying atherosclerosis, (2) the extent and type of thrombus that forms over the ruptured plaque, (3) the degree and extent of coronary vasospasm, and (4) the underlying myocardial substrate. The degree of coronary artery luminal stenosis does not correlate well with acute cardiac events, and most myocardial infarctions occur at sites with less than 50% luminal stenosis [82]. Whether patients present clinically with unstable angina, non–ST-segment elevation myocardial infarction, or ST-segment elevation myocardial infarction is dependent on the degree and duration of the occlusion and the amount of myocardium that sustains infarction as a result of the occlusion. In unstable angina, the occlusions and episodes of ischemia are brief and myocardial cell necrosis does not occur. In non–ST-segment elevation myocardial infarction, the episodes of ischemia and occlusions are more prolonged and myocardial necrosis occurs. The resultant necrosis does not usually extend to the full thickness of the myocardium. In ST-segment elevation myocardial infarction (previously referred to as Q wave infarction), the occlusion produces necrosis that usually extends through the full thickness of the myocardium.

Acute coronary syndromes in African Americans

Although there is great interest in the possible significance of differences that have been reported in CHD manifestations and outcomes between blacks and whites, considerable confusion and controversy remain. The clinical spectrum of African Americans presenting with ACSs is the same as for white patients presenting with ACSs; however, African Americans more often have non–ST-segment elevation syndromes (sudden death, non–Q wave infarction, or unstable angina) and have poorer outcomes than whites [83,84]. The reasons for these findings have not been fully elucidated but may be related to (1) the greater prevalence and severity of certain risk factors, particularly hypertension and its consequences in African Americans; (2) excessive delays in seeking medical care by African Americans and later presentation in the clinical evolution of ACSs; (3) delays in diagnosis of ACSs in African Americans who present to emergency departments with chest pain; and (4) less aggressive medical and interventional therapies (cardiac catheterization, percutaneous coronary interventions, and bypass surgery) following confirmation of ACSs.

Prehospital delay

African Americans delay seeking medical care for ACSs and present later (up to three times longer) in their clinical course than whites [85–88]. It has been well studied and documented that greater benefits are achieved (eg, infarct size reduction, mortality) when therapy is initiated earlier in the course of ACSs. Delays in seeking medical care limit these benefits and contribute to increased morbidity and mortality. Many factors contribute to health care–seeking behavior, including access to medical care, knowledge and beliefs concerning CHD, symptom perception, and attributions and adherence to treatment recommendations. Access to medical care is an important contributor to delays because patients without a usual care provider, patients of low socioeconomic strata, and patients with poor insurance coverage delay seeking care for acute events.

Although much of the treatment delay for ACSs has been attributed to delayed seeking of medical care and delayed initial hospital arrival following onset of symptoms, substantial treatment delays may also occur between the time the patient arrives in the hospital and initiation of definitive therapy. Because African-American patients present later in the clinical course of their ACSs and are at higher risk, there should be a greater urgency in terms of timely evaluation, diagnosis, risk assessment, and treatment. Paradoxically, the opposite is true.

Emergency room presentation and initial evaluation

Most African-American patients (70%–85%) who have myocardial ischemia and acute myocardial infarction present with chest pain, although African Americans who have acute myocardial ischemia have been reported to have more atypical symptoms than their white counterparts [89–94]. In the emergency department, the index of suspicion for coronary ischemia is often lower for African Americans than it is for whites [94], and symptoms are less often attributed to coronary disease by patients and by the providers who initially evaluate them [94]. Perhaps as a consequence, first ECGs are performed later in African Americans than in whites, and physicians perform laboratory evaluation (cardiac markers) and noninvasive and invasive diagnostics to evaluate for coronary disease less often in African Americans than in whites. Even when myocardial ischemia is suspected during the initial evaluation, nonspecific or nondiagnostic repolarization abnormalities on ECG may make the diagnosis of ischemia or myocardial infarction difficult.

Optimal approach to patients who have acute coronary syndromes

The optimal approach to the management of ACSs continues to evolve, and in-hospital outcomes in patients who have ACSs continue to improve. Early, complete, and sustained reperfusion using thrombolytic therapy or percutaneous coronary interventions is the primary goal of treatment in patients who have ST-segment elevation myocardial infarction [95]. The management of patients who have non–ST-segment elevation myocardial infarction or unstable angina is more challenging and requires careful integration of overall risk assessment and pharmacologic and interventional/mechanical therapies [96].

One of the guiding principles for management of patients who have ACSs is that the intensity of therapy should be based on the overall risk, with patients at highest risk receiving the most immediate and intensive therapy [97–99]. The goals of initial treatment in patients who have ACSs include relief of angina, control of the acute aspects of the pathophysiologic processes, preservation of viable myocardium, and prevention of death. Initial treatments strategies include antithrombotic and antiplatelet therapy, antianginal medications, mechanical revascularization, and pharmacologic measures to stabilize plaques and modify risk factors. Accurate diagnosis and risk stratification are essential for appropriate therapy because patients who have ACSs are heterogeneous and exhibit varying degrees of risk for death and recurrent ischemic events. Several clinical risk models have been developed to help classify patients into low-, moderate/intermediate-, and high-risk groups. One such risk stratification tool is the Thrombolysis in Myocardial Infarction (TIMI) risk score [97], which effectively predicts prognosis in patients who have ACSs and is a useful tool for helping to select appropriate therapeutic strategies. The TIMI risk score was developed and validated using the database of the TIMI 11B trial [97]. Although very useful, the TIMI risk score has not yet been validated in African Americans.

In high-risk ACS patients, an invasive strategy (early angiography and revascularization) is the preferred approach when it is available and accessible in a timely manner; however, invasive and conservative (medical) approaches should be considered complementary. Modern aggressive protocol–driven medical therapy may decrease cardiac ischemia, cardiac events, and the urgency for revascularization. Early angiography and revascularization strategies play a particularly important role in the management of patients who belong to higher risk categories.

Treatment of acute coronary syndromes in African Americans

Based on higher risk status and poorer outcomes, it would appear that African Americans who have ACSs should be treated at least as aggressively as and perhaps more aggressively than whites; however, this is not the case, and African-American patients who have ACSs paradoxically receive less aggressive medical therapy and are less likely to receive reperfusion therapies such as thrombolytics and undergo coronary revascularization procedures [100–117]. The reasons for this treatment disparity are unclear but have been attributed to unmeasured confounders that may impact the process of care for black patients (such as hospital characteristics, physician and patient preferences, and cultural and socioeconomic factors) and possible physician bias in the use of aggressive thrombolytic therapies and invasive cardiac procedures.

At the time of presentation, African Americans who have ACSs are more likely than whites to have comorbidities (hypertension, diabetes, renal insufficiency, history of heart failure, smoking) that might lead clinicians to select a more conservative treatment strategy, but even after adjustments for baseline characteristics, blacks receive thrombolysis, angiography, percutaneous coronary interventions, and bypass surgery less often.

Diagnosis, risk assessment, and prevention of coronary heart disease

Diagnosis and risk assessment

Although generally not difficult, the accurate diagnosis of CHD in African Americans may present special challenges. The higher prevalence of hypertension and type 2 diabetes mellitus may contribute to discordance between symptomatology and the presence of obstructive coronary disease. Many commonly accepted diagnostic modalities used for risk assessment have not been validated in African Americans, and some appear to have a lower predictive value in African Americans. Individuals with hypertension and hypertensive heart disease may have ischemic chest pain in the absence of obstructive coronary disease. In the Framingham Heart Study, hypertensive patients were more likely to have unrecognized myocardial infarction than nonhypertensive patients [118]. The high prevalence of type 2 diabetes mellitus in African Americans may further predispose these individuals to silent ischemia or atypical symptoms.

Nondiagnostic ST-segment and T wave changes, early repolarization changes, and increased QRS wave voltage on ECG are more common in African-American men than in white men. These ECG abnormalities are often interpreted as "normal variants"; however, their role as markers of increased CHD risk for African Americans has not been evaluated. In contrast, ECG may assist in defining the possible contributions of hypertension and left ventricular hypertrophy to the clinical manifestations and natural history of CHD in African Americans.

The interpretation of exercise ECG tests in African Americans may be unreliable because of the high frequency of baseline ST-segment and T wave abnormalities.

Exercise testing with myocardial imaging (thallium and other radio-isotopes) may provide better diagnostic accuracy; however, the presence of underlying hypertensive heart disease can result in a high rate of false-positive results. More recent diagnostic modalities for the evaluation of myocardial ischemia and function (ie, positron emission tomography, MRI, magnetic resonance angiography, and intravascular ultrasound) are promising. Their diagnostic accuracy and role in the risk assessment of African Americans have not been determined. Likewise, the predictive value of coronary calcification by digital subtraction fluoroscopy in African Americans remains to be established.

Primary and secondary prevention

The high CHD morbidity and mortality rates in African Americans can be largely accounted for by the high prevalence of CHD risk factors. Many of these risk factors are modifiable and thus prevent opportunities for primary and secondary prevention. Primary prevention refers to the prevention of coronary disease and coronary events in individuals who do not have disease and provides the greatest opportunity for reducing CHD morbidity and mortality. This approach focuses primarily on lifestyle modifications (diet, increased physical activity, weight control, and avoidance of lifestyles such as smoking that adversely impact risk). Secondary prevention refers to reduction of total mortality, coronary mortality, major coronary events, need for coronary procedures, and stroke in individuals who have established CHD. Individuals who do not have established CHD but are at high risk (ie, patients who have diabetes) are considered to have CHD equivalents and require the same intensity of treatment and risk reduction as those who have known CHD.

Therapeutic lifestyle changes

All modifiable risk factors should be approached vigorously. Patients who smoke cigarettes should be urged to stop and assisted in doing so. Dietary modification is the cornerstone of therapy for patients who have hypercholesterolemia, hypertension, obesity, diabetes mellitus, and the metabolic syndrome. The principles of dietary modification for each of these disorders are similar and include reducing the intake of calories, saturated fat, total fat, cholesterol, and alcohol. Weight reduction and control and increased physical activity are also essential for effective management. Even limited weight loss is often helpful. It is important to remind patients that weight reduction and control are long-term rather than short-term therapies and that success is achieved only through long-term lifestyle modifications that emphasize nutritional balance and physical activity. Moderate exercise helps in losing weight, lowering cholesterol, reducing hyperinsulinemia (even without weight loss), lowering blood pressure, improving cardiovascular fitness, and decreasing overall cardiovascular risk.

Pharmacologic therapy

In individuals with incomplete responses to diet, exercise, and other therapeutic lifestyle changes, drug therapy to specifically reduce selected cardiovascular risk factors should be considered. The benefits of treating atherogenic dyslpidemia and lowering blood pressure are well established [40,119]. In addition, aspirin (81–160 mg daily) is recommended for adults at intermediate risk for CHD events for treatment of the prothrombotic state (prevention of CHD and stroke) [120]. Although the benefits of treatment of hyperglycemia to reduce CHD and stroke risk have not yet been established, tight control of fasting and postprandial glucose levels and HbA_{1C} is recommended. Drug therapies that reduce insulin resistance are available, but there is no evidence as yet that they reduce the risk of CHD [121].

Improving patient compliance with therapy

A major barrier to CHD prevention is lack of patient compliance with therapy. Important contributors to lack of compliance include problems with doctor–patient communications, cost, and medication side effects [40,122]. Poor communication between physicians and patients may be the most important impediment to effective adherence to treatment. Improvement in physician–patient interaction requires mutual participation and commitment (Box 3). Physicians must convey interest in controlling the patient's risk factors and a commitment to overcoming obstacles. Physicians must spend time educating patients about the importance of risk factor control, taking their medications, and the goals of therapy. Patient responsibilities include keeping follow-up appointments, following non-pharmacologic recommendations, and alerting the physician to other

---

Box 3. Guidelines for improving compliance with antihypertensive and lipid-lowering therapy

Physician's role
- Convey interest and commitment to controlling patient's blood pressure and dyslipidemia
- Educate/communicate to patient importance of treatment, control, and achieving goals
- Tell patient his/her blood pressure and cholesterol levels at each visit
- Provide written reminders of appointments
- Ask patient specifically about drug side effects
- Relate medication taking to other daily activities
- Avoid miscommunication (achievement of goal blood pressure and lipid levels does not mean cure or that medication can be stopped)
- Inform patient of mutual responsibility in achieving treatment goals

Patient's role
- Accept commitment to achieve blood pressure and cholesterol control
- Keep follow-up appointments
- Follow all therapeutic lifestyle change recommendations (weight control, physical activity, salt intake, and so forth)
- Alert physician to any problem with medications (eg, side effects, scheduling conflicts, problem with costs)

prescribed medications or problems with medicines. Patients infrequently volunteer cost as a reason for failure to take medications or keep follow-up appointments, and few report discontinuing medications because they cannot afford them. Cost, however, is a more frequent impediment to effective therapy than is generally appreciated. Patients who have hypertension, dyslipidemia, the metabolic syndrome, and certain other risk factors are often asymptomatic. Therefore, the impact of therapy on quality of life is an important concern, and treatments that contribute to a feeling of unwellness reduce adherence to therapy. The effects of treatment on patients' quality of life—emotional, physical, cognitive, and social functioning—should be monitored, and patients must be put on therapeutic regimens that minimally affect these parameters if effective control is to be achieved.

Prevention for children

The epidemic of obesity in adults in the United States has been accompanied by an increase in the proportion of children who are overweight [42] due to an increase in caloric intake and a decrease in physical activity. Thus, it is important that preventive measures focus on adults and children. Individual measures to decrease sedentary lifestyles (eg, less television hours, and so forth) are extremely important, as are community and public health measures (eg, increasing the number and safety of walking areas, eliminating high-calorie fast-food specials, providing simple nutrition information on food labels, increasing school-based physical activity programs, and other measures).

Summary

Cardiovascular disease (in particular, CHD) is the leading cause of death in the United States for Americans of both sexes and of all racial and ethnic backgrounds. African Americans have the highest overall CHD mortality rate and the highest out-of-hospital coronary death rate of any ethnic group in the United States, particularly at younger ages. Contributors to the earlier onset of CHD and excess CHD deaths among African Americans include a high prevalence of coronary risk factors, patient delays in seeking medical care, and disparities in health care.

The clinical spectrum of acute and chronic CHD in African Americans is the same as in whites; however, African Americans have a higher risk of sudden cardiac death and present clinically more often with unstable angina and non–ST-segment elevation myocardial infarction than whites. Although generally not difficult, the accurate diagnosis and risk assessment for CHD in African Americans may at times present special challenges. The high prevalence of hypertension and type 2 diabetes mellitus may contribute to discordance between symptomatology and the severity of coronary artery disease, and some noninvasive tests appear to have a lower predictive value for disease.

Box 4. Essentials for improving outcomes and reducing cardiovascular disease disparities

More education and advocacy to increase provider and public awareness of disparities

Aggressive treatment of all modifiable risk factors (hypertension, dyslipidemia, obesity, physical inactivity, smoking)

Targeting of high-risk patients (ie, those who have multiple risk factors, the metabolic syndrome, left ventricular hypertrophy, diabetes mellitus) for intensive risk-reduction measures

Decreasing patient delays in seeking medical care for acute myocardial infarction and other cardiac disorders

More timely and appropriate therapy for ACSs

More effective implementation of evidence-based treatment guidelines

Improved access to preventive, diagnostic, and interventional cardiovascular therapies

Improved physician–patient communications

The high prevalence of modifiable risk factors provides great opportunities for the prevention of CHD in African Americans. Patients at high risk should be targeted for intensive risk reduction measures, early recognition/ diagnosis of ischemic syndromes, and appropriate referral for coronary interventions and cardiac surgical procedures. African Americans who have ACSs receive less aggressive treatment than their white counterparts but they should not. Use of evidence-based therapies for management of patients who have ACSs and better understanding of various available treatment strategies are of utmost importance.

Reducing and ultimately eliminating disparities in cardiovascular care and outcomes require comprehensive programs of education and advocacy (Box 4) with the goals of (1) increasing provider and public awareness of the disparities in treatment; (2) decreasing patient delays in seeking medical care for acute myocardial infarction and other cardiac disorders; (3) more timely and appropriate therapy for ACSs; (4) improved access to preventive, diagnostic, and interventional cardiovascular therapies; (5) more effective implementation of evidence-based treatment guidelines; and (6) improved physician–patient communications.

References

[1] American Heart Association. Heart disease and stroke statistics—2005 update. Available at: http://www.americanheart.org. Accessed March 14, 2005.

[2] Anderson R, Smith B. Deaths: leading causes for 2001. National Vital Statistics Reports, vol. 52, no. 9. Hyattsville (MD): National Center for Health Statistics; 2003.

[3] Gillum RF. Coronary heart disease in black populations I: mortality and morbidity. Am Heart J 1982;104:839–51.

[4] Gillum RF, Graham CT. Coronary heart disease in black populations II: risk factors. Am Heart J 1982;104:852–64.

[5] Clark LT, Ferdinand KC, Flack JM, et al. Coronary heart disease in African Americans. Heart Dis 2001;3:97–108.

[6] Centers for Disease Control and Prevention (CDC). Disparities in premature deaths from heart disease—50 states and the District of Columbia, 2001. MMWR Morb Mortal Wkly Rep 2004;53:121–5.

[7] Francis CK, Grant AO, cochairs. Report of the Working Group on Research in Coronary Heart Disease in Blacks. Washington DC: National Institutes of Health, US Department of Health and Human Services; 1994.

[8] Traven N, Kuller L, Ives D. Coronary heart disease mortality and sudden death among the 35–44 year age group in Allegheny County, Pennsylvania. Ann Epidemiol 1996;6:130–6.

[9] Gillium R, Mussolino M, Madans J. Coronary heart disease incidence and survival in African-American women and men. The NHANES I epidemiologic follow-up study. Ann Intern Med 1997;127:111–8.

[10] Gillium R. Sudden cardiac death in Hispanic Americans and African Americans. Am J Public Health 1997;87:1461–6.

[11] Clark LT. Anatomic substrate differences between black and white victims of sudden cardiac death: hypertension, coronary artery disease or both? Clin Cardiol 1989;12(Suppl IV):IV13–7.

[12] National Medical Association History. Available at: http://www.nmanet.org/History.htm. Accessed March 14, 2005.

[13] Stone CT, Vanzant FR. Heart disease as seen in a southern clinic: clinical and pathological survey. JAMA 1927;89:1473–7.

[14] US Department of Health and Human Services. Report of the Secretary's Task Force on Black and Minority Health, vol. 4: cardiovascular and cerebrovascular diseases. Washington, DC: US Department of Health and Human Services; 1986.

[15] Smedley BD, Stith AY, Nelson AR, editors. Committee on Understanding and Eliminating Racial and Ethnic Disparities in Health Care. Unequal treatment: confronting racial and ethnic disparities in health care. Washington, DC: The National Academies Press; 2003.

[16] The Henry J. Kaiser Family Foundation and American College of Cardiology Foundation. Racial/ethnic differences in cardiac care: the weight of the evidence summary report. Menlo Park (CA): The Henry J. Kaiser Family Foundation and American College of Cardiology Foundation; 2002.

[17] Rowland ML, Fulwood R. Coronary heart disease risk factor trends in blacks between the First and Second National Health and Nutrition Examination Surveys, United States, 1971–1980. Am Heart J 1984;108:771–9.

[18] Cutter GR, Burke GL, Dyer AR, et al. Cardiovascular risk factors in young adults. The CARDIA baseline monograph. Control Clin Trials 1991;12:1S–77S.

[19] Hutchinson RG, Watson RL, Davis CE, et al. Racial differences in risk factors for atherosclerosis. The ARIC study. Angiology 1997;48:279–90.

[20] Neaton JD, Kuller LH, Wentworth D, et al. Total and cardiovascular mortality in relation to cigarette smoking, serum cholesterol concentration, and diastolic blood pressure among black and white males followed up for five years. Am Heart J 1984;108:759–69.

[21] Cooper RS, Liao Y, Rotimi C. Is hypertension more severe among US blacks, or is severe hypertension more common? Ann Epidemiol 1996;6:173–80.

[22] Liao Y, Cooper RS, McGee DL, et al. The relative effects of left ventricular hypertrophy, coronary artery disease, and ventricular dysfunction on survival among black adults. JAMA 1995;273:1592–7.

[23] Gavin JR III. Diabetes in minorities: reflections on the medical dilemma and the healthcare crisis. Trans Am Clin Climatol Assoc 1995;107:213–23.

[24] Moliterno DJ, Jokinen EV, Miserez AR, et al. No association between plasma lipoprotein(a) concentrations and the presence or absence of coronary atherosclerosis in African-Americans. Arterioscler Thromb Vasc Biol 1995;15:850–5.

[25] Guyton JR, Dahlen GH, Patsch W, et al. Relationship of plasma lipoprotein Lp(a) levels to race and to apolipoprotein B. Arteriosclerosis 1985;5:265–72.

[26] Sorrentino MJ, Vielhauer C, Eisenbart JD, et al. Plasma lipoprotein(a) protein concentration and coronary artery disease in black patients compared with white patients. Am J Med 1992;93:658–62.

[27] Schreiner PJ, Heiss G, Tyroler HA, et al. Race and gender differences in the association of Lp(a) with carotid artery wall thickness. The Atherosclerosis Risk in Communities (ARIC) study. Arterioscler Thromb Vasc Biol 1996;16:471–8.

[28] Saunders E. Hypertension in African-Americans. Circulation 1991;83:1465–7.

[29] Jamerson KA. Geographical aspects of hypertension. Prevalence of complications and response to different treatments of hypertension in African Americans and white Americans in the US. Clin Exp Hypertens 1993;15:979–95.

[30] Rahman M, Douglas JG, Wright JT Jr. Pathophysiology and treatment implications of hypertension in the African-American population. Endocrinol Metab Clin N Am 1997;26: 125–44.

[31] Chobanian AV, Bakris GL, Black HR, et al. Joint National Committee on Prevention, Detection, Evaluation, and Treatment of High Blood Pressure. National Heart, Lung, and Blood Institute; National High Blood Pressure Education Program Coordinating Committee. Seventh report of the Joint National Committee on Prevention, Detection, Evaluation, and Treatment of High Blood Pressure. JAMA 2003;289:2560–71.

[32] Douglas JG, Bakris GL, Epstein M, et al. Management of high blood pressure in African Americans: consensus statement of the Hypertension in African Americans Working Group of the International Society on Hypertension in Blacks. Arch Intern Med 2003;163: 525–41.

[33] Harris MI, Flegal KM, Cowie CC, et al. Prevalence of diabetes, impaired fasting glucose, and impaired glucose tolerance in US adults. The Third National Health and Nutrition Examination Survey, 1988–1994. Diabetes Care 1998;21:518–24.

[34] Carter JS, Pugh JA, Monterrosa A. Non–insulin-dependent diabetes mellitus in minorities in the United States. Ann Intern Med 1996;125:221–32.

[35] Folsom AR, Szklo M, Stevens J, et al. A prospective study of coronary heart disease in relation to fasting insulin, glucose, and diabetes. The Atherosclerosis Risk in Communities (ARIC) study. Diabetes Care 1997;20:935–42.

[36] Chin MH, Zhang JX, Merrell K. Diabetes in the African-American Medicare population. Morbidity, quality of care, and resource utilization. Diabetes Care 1998;21:1090–5.

[37] Haffner SM. Epidemiology of type 2 diabetes: risk factors. Diabetes Care 1998;21(Suppl 3): C3–6.

[38] Brancati FL, Kao WHL, Folsom AR, et al. Incident type 2 diabetes mellitus in African American and white adults. The Atherosclerosis Risk in Communities study. JAMA 2000; 283:2253–9.

[39] Bonds DE, Zaccaro DJ, Karter AJ, et al. Ethnic and racial differences in diabetes care: the Insulin Resistance Atherosclerosis Study. Diabetes Care 2003;26:1040–6.

[40] Grundy SM, Becker D, Clark LT, et al. Third Report of the National Cholesterol Education Program (NCEP) Expert Panel on Detection, Evaluation, and Treatment of High Blood Cholesterol in Adults (Adult Treatment Panel III). Final report. Circulation 2002;106:3145–421.

[41] Ford ES, Giles WH, Dietz WH. Prevalence of the metabolic syndrome among US adults: findings from the Third National Health and Nutritional Examination Survey. JAMA 2002;287:356–9.

[42] Hall WD, Clark LT, Wenger NK, et al. The metabolic syndrome in African Americans: a review. Ethn Dis 2003;13:414–28.

[43] Wong ND, Pio JR, Franklin SS, et al. Preventing coronary events by optimal control of blood pressure and lipids in patients with the metabolic syndrome. Am J Cardiol 2003;91: 1421–6.

[44] Brunzell JD, Hokanson JE. Dyslipidemia of central obesity and insulin resistance. Diabetes Care 1999;22:C10–3.

[45] Bjorntorp P. Body fat distribution, insulin resistance, and metabolic diseases. Nutrition 1997;13:795–803.

[46] Bonow RO. Primary prevention of cardiovascular disease: a call to action. Circulation 2002;106:3140–1.

[47] Flegal KM, Carroll MD, Ogden CL, et al. Prevalence and trends in obesity among US adults, 1999–2000. JAMA 2002;288:1723–7.

[48] Flegal KM, Carroll MD, Kuczmarski RJ, et al. Overweight and obesity in the United States: prevalence and trends, 1960–1994. Int J Obes Relat Metab Disord 1998;22: 39–47.

[49] Perry AC, Applegate EB, Jackson ML, et al. Racial differences in visceral adipose tissue but not anthropometric markers of health-related variables. J Appl Physiol 2000;89:636–43.

[50] Donahue RP, Jacobs DR Jr, Sidney S, et al. Distribution of lipoproteins and apolipoproteins in young adults. The CARDIA Study. Arteriosclerosis 1989;9:656–64.

[51] Watkins LO, Neaton JD, Kuller LH. Racial differences in high-density lipoprotein cholesterol and coronary heart disease incidence in the usual care group of the Multiple Risk Factor Intervention Trial. Am J Cardiol 1986;57:538–45.

[52] Sprafka JM, Burke GL, Folsom AR, et al. Hypercholesterolemia prevalence, awareness, and treatment in blacks and whites: the Minnesota Heart Survey. Prev Med 1989;18: 423–32.

[53] Gidding SS, Liu K, Bild DE, et al. Prevalence and identification of abnormal lipoprotein levels in a biracial population aged 23 to 35 years (the CARDIA study). The Coronary Risk Development in Young Adults study. Am J Cardiol 1996;78:304–8.

[54] Boden WE. High-density lipoprotein cholesterol as an independent risk factor in cardiovascular disease: assessing the data from Framingham to the Veterans Affairs High-Density Lipoprotein Intervention Trial. Am J Cardiol 2000;86:19L–22L.

[55] Vega GL, Clark LT, Tang A, et al. Hepatic lipase activity is lower in African American men than in white American men: effects of 5′ flanking polymorphism in the hepatic lipase gene (LIPC). J Lipid Res 1998;39:228–32.

[56] Austin MA, Hokanson JE, Edwards KL. Hypertriglyceridemia as a cardiovascular risk factor. Am J Cardiol 1998;81(4A):7B–12B.

[57] Watson KE, Topol EJ. Pathobiology of atherosclerosis: are there racial and ethnic differences? Rev Cardiovasc Med 2004;5(Suppl 3):S14–21.

[58] Centers for Disease Control and Prevention. Prevalence of cigarette use among 14 racial/ ethnic populations—United Status, 1999–2001. MMWR Morb Mortal Wkly Rep 2004;53: 49–52.

[59] Okuyemi KS, Ebersole-Robinson M, Nazir N, et al. African-American menthol and nonmenthol smokers: differences in smoking and cessation experiences. J Natl Med Assoc 2004;96(9):1208–11.

[60] Sesso HD, Paffenbarger RS, Lee I. Physical activity and coronary heart disease in men. Circulation 2000;102:975.

[61] Thompson PD, Buchner D, Pina IL, et al. Exercise and physical activity in the prevention and treatment of atherosclerotic cardiovascular disease: a statement from the Council on Clinical Cardiology (Subcommittee on Exercise, Rehabilitation, and Prevention) and the Council on Nutrition, Physical Activity, and Metabolism (Subcommittee on Physical Activity). Circulation 2003;107:3109–16.

[62] Ross R. Atherosclerosis—an inflammatory disease. N Engl J Med 1999;340:115–26.

[63] Clark LT. Vascular inflammation as a therapeutic target for prevention of cardiovascular disease. Curr Atheroscler Rep 2002;4:77–81.

[64] Albert MA, Torres J, Glynn RJ, et al. Perspective on selected issues in cardiovascular disease research with a focus on black Americans. Circulation 2004;110:e7–12.

[65] Stone PH, Thompson B, Anderson HV, et al, for the TIMI III Registry Study Group. Influence of race, sex and age on management of unstable angina and non-Q-wave myocardial infarction. JAMA 1996;275:1104–12.

[66] Simmons BE, Castaner A, Campo A, et al. Coronary artery disease in blacks of lower socioeconomic status: angiographic findings from the Cook Country Hospital Heart Disease Registry. Am Heart J 1989;116:90–7.

[67] Maynard C, Fisher LD, Passamani ER. Survival of black persons compared with white persons in the Coronary Artery Surgery Study (CASS). Am J Cardiol 1987;60:513–8.

[68] Thomas J, Thomas DJ, Pearson T, et al. Cardiovascular disease in African- American and white physicians: the Meharry Cohort and Meharry-Hopkins Cohort Studies. J Health Care Poor Underserved 1997;8:270–83.

[69] Strong JP, Malcom GT, Oalmann MC, et al. The PDAY study: natural history, risk factors, and pathobiology. Pathobiological Determinants of Atherosclerosis in Youth. Ann N Y Acad Sci 1997;811:226–35.

[70] Davies MJ. The role of plaque pathology in coronary thrombosis. Clin Cardiol 1997; 20(Suppl I):I2–7.

[71] Fuster V. Acute coronary syndromes: the degree and morphology of coronary stenoses. J Am Coll Cardiol 2000;35:52B–4B.

[72] Falk E, Shah PK, Fuster V. Coronary plaque disruption. Circulation 1995;92:657–71.

[73] Selwyn AP, Kinlay S, Creager M, et al. Cell dysfunction in atherosclerosis and the ischemic manifestations of coronary artery disease. Am J Cardiol 1997;79:17–23.

[74] Glasser SP, Selwyn AP, Ganz P. Atherosclerosis: risk factors and the vascular endothelium. Am Heart J 1996;131:379–84.

[75] Gibbons GH. Endothelial function as a determinant of vascular function and structure: a new therapeutic target. Am J Cardiol 1997;79:3–8.

[76] Takase B, Uehata A, Akima A, et al. Endothelium-dependent flow-mediated vasodilation in coronary and brachial arteries in suspected coronary artery disease. Am J Cardiol 1998; 82:1535–9.

[77] Treasure CB, Klein JL, Vita JA, et al. Hypertension and left ventricular hypertrophy are associated with impaired endothelium-mediated relaxation in human coronary resistance vessels. Circulation 1993;87:86–93.

[78] Tsurumi Y, Nagashima H, Ichikawa K, et al. Influence of plasma lipoprotein(a) levels on coronary vasomotor response to acetylcholine. J Am Coll Cardiol 1995;26:1242–50.

[79] Houghton JL, Smith VE, Strogatz DS, et al. Effect of African-American race and hypertensive left ventricular hypertrophy on coronary vascular reactivity and endothelial function. Hypertension 1997;29:706–14.

[80] Houghton JL, Davison CA, Kuhner PA, et al. Heterogeneous vasomotor responses of coronary conduit and resistance vessels in hypertension. J Am Coll Cardiol 1998;31:374–82.

[81] Ergul S, Parish DC, Puett D, et al. Racial differences in plasma endothelin-1 concentrations in individuals with essential hypertension. Hypertension 1996;28:652–5.

[82] Ambrose JA, Fuster V. The risk of coronary occlusion is not proportional to the prior severity of coronary stenosis. Heart 1998;79:3–4.

[83] Nakamura Y, Moss AJ, Brown MW, et al. Ethnicity and long-term outcome after an acute coronary event. Multicenter Myocardial Ischemia Research Group. Am Heart J 1999;138: 500–6.

[84] Asher CR, Topol EJ, Moliterno DJ. Insights into the pathophysiology of atherosclerosis prognosis of black Americans who have acute coronary syndromes. Am Heart J 1999;138: 1073–81.

[85] Clark LT, Bellam SV, Shah AH, et al. Analysis of prehospital delay among inner-city patients with symptoms of myocardial infarction: implications for the therapeutic intervention. J Natl Med Assc 1992;84:931–7.

[86] Cooper RS, Simmons B, Castaner A, et al. Survival rates and prehospital delay during myocardial infarction among black persons. Am J Cardiol 1986;57:208–11.

[87] Crawford SL, McGraw SA, Smith KW, et al. Do blacks and whites differ in their use of health care for symptoms of coronary heart disease? Am J Public Health 1994;84:957–64.

[88] Dracup K, Moser DK, Eisenberg M, et al. Causes of delay in seeking treatment for heart attack symptoms. Soc Sci Med 1995;40:379–92.

[89] Summers RL, Cooper GJ, Carlton FB, et al. Prevalence of atypical chest pain descriptions in a population from the southern United States. Am J Med Sci 1999;318:142–5.

[90] Ghali JK, Cooper RS, Kowatly I, et al. Delay between onset of chest pain and arrival to the coronary care unit among minority and disadvantaged patients. J Natl Med Assoc 1993;85: 180–4.

[91] Johnson PA, Lee TH, Cook EF, et al. Effect of race on the presentation and management of patients with acute chest pain. Ann Inten Med 1993;118:593–601.

[92] Taylor HA Jr, Canto JG, Sanderson B, et al. Mangement and outcomes for black patients with acute myocardial infarction in the reperfusion era. Am J Cardiol 1998;82:1019–23.

[93] Raczynski JM, Taylor H, Cutter G, et al. Diagnoses, symptoms, and attribution of symptoms among black and white inpatients admitted for coronary heart disease. Am J Public Health 1994;84:951–6.

[94] Venkat A, Hoekstra J, Lindsell C, et al. The impact of race on the acute management of chest pain. Acad Emerg Med 2003;10:1199–208.

[95] Ryan T, Antman E, Brooks N, et al. 1999 update: ACC/AHA guidelines for the management of patients with acute myocardial infarction. J Am Coll Cardiol 1999;34: 889–911.

[96] Braunwald E, Antman E, Beasley J, et al. ACC/AHA 2002 guideline update for the management of patients with unstable angina and non-ST-segment elevation myocardial infarction. J Am Coll Cardiol 2002;40(7):1366–74.

[97] Cannon C, Weintraub W, Demopoulos L, et al. Comparison of early invasive and conservative strategies in patients with unstable coronary syndromes treated with the glycoprotein IIb/IIIa inhibitor tirofiban (TACTICS-TIMI 18). N Engl J Med 2001;344(25): 1879–87.

[98] The FRISCII Investigators. Invasive compared with non-invasive treatment in unstable coronary artery disease: FRISC II prospective randomized multicenter study. Lancet 1999; 354:708–15.

[99] Fox K, Poole-Wilson P, Henderon R, et al. Interventional versus conservative treatment for patients with unstable angina or non-ST-elevation myocardial infarction: the British Heart Foundation RITA 3 randomized trial. Randomized Intervention Trial of Unstable Angina. Lancet 2002;360:743–51.

[100] Leape LL, Hilborne LH, Bell R, et al. Underuse of cardiac procedures: do women, ethnic minorities, and the uninsured fail to receive needed revascularization? Ann Intern Med 1999;130:183–92.

[101] Scirica BM, Molitterno DJ, Every NR, et al, for the GUARANTEE Investigators. Racial differences in the management of unstable angina: results from the multicenter GUARANTEE registry. Am Heart J 1999;138:1065–72.

[102] Weitzman S, Cooper L, Chamblesss L, et al. Gender, racial, and geographic differences in the performance of cardiac diagnostic and therapeutic procedures for hospitalized acute myocardial infarction in four states. Am J Cardiol 1997;79:722–6.

[103] Gillum RF, Gillum BS, Francis CK. Coronary revascularization and cardiac catheterization in the United States: trends in racial differences. J Am Coll Cardiol 1997;29:1557–62.

[104] Peterson ED, Shaw LK, DeLong ER, et al. Racial variation in the use of coronary-revascularization procedures. Are the differences real? Do they matter? N Engl J Med 1997; 336:480–6.

[105] Gillum RF. Coronary artery bypass surgery and coronary angiography in the United States, 1979–1983. Am Heart J 1987;113:1255–60.

[106] Ford ES, Cooper RS. Racial/ethnic differences in health care utilization of cardiovascular procedures: a review of the evidence. Health Serv Res 1995;30:237–52.

[107] Maynard C, Litwin PE, Martin JS, et al. Characteristics of black patients admitted to coronary care units in metropolitan Seattle: results from the Myocardial Infarction Triage and Intervention Registry (MITI). Am J Cardiol 1991;67:18–23.

[108] Hannan EL, Kilburn H, O'Donnell JF, et al. Interracial access to selected cardiac procedures for the patients hospitalized with coronary artery disease in New York State. Med Care 1991;29:430–41.

[109] Mirvis DM, Burns R, Gaschen L, et al. Variation in utilization of cardiac procedures in the Department of Veterans Affairs health care system: effect of race. J Am Coll Cardiol 1994; 24:1297–304.

[110] National Heart, Lung, and Blood Institute. Proceedings of the conference on Socioeconomic Status and Cardiovascular Health and Disease, November 6–7, 1995. Bethesda (MD): National Institute of Health; 1995.

[111] Diez-Roux AV, Nieto FJ, Tyroler HN, et al. Social inequalities and atherosclerosis. The Atherosclerosis Risk in Communities study. Am J Epidemiol 1995;141:960–72.

[112] Dracup K, Moser DK. Treatment-seeking behavior among those with signs and symptoms of acute myocardial infarction. Heart Lung 1991;20:570–5.

[113] Taylor AJ, Meyer GS, Morse RW, et al. Can characteristics of a health care system mitigate ethnic bias in access to cardiovascular procedures? Experience from the Military Health Services system. J Am Coll Cardiol 1997;30:901–7.

[114] Ferguson JA, Tierney WM, Westmoreland GR, et al. Examination of racial differences in the management of cardiovascular disease. J Am Coll Cardiol 1997;30:1707–13.

[115] Harris DR, Andrews R, Elixhauser A. Racial and gender differences in use of procedures for black and white hospitalized adults. Ethn Dis 1997;7:91–105.

[116] Wu AH, Parsons L, Every NR, et al. Hospital outcomes in patients presenting with congestive heart failure complicating acute myocardial infarction: a report from the Second National Registry of Myocardial Infarction (NRMI-2). J Am Coll Cardiol 2002;40: 1389–94.

[117] Sonel AF, Good CB, Mulgund J, et al, for the CRUSADE Investigators Racial Variations in Treatment and Outcomes of Black and White Patients with High-Risk Non–ST-Elevation Acute Coronary Syndromes. Insights from CRUSADE (Can Rapid Risk Stratification of Unstable Angina Patients Suppress Adverse Outcomes with Early Implementation of the ACC/AHA Guidelines?). Circulation 2005;111:1225–32.

[118] Kannel WB, Abbott RD, Dannenberg AL, et al. The PDAY study: natural history, risk factors, and pathobiology. Pathobiological Determinants of Atherosclerosis in Youth. Ann N Y Acad Sci 1997;811:226–35.

[119] Grundy SM, Cleeman JI, Merz CN, et al. National Heart, Lung, and Blood Institute; American College of Cardiology Foundation; American Heart Association. Implications of recent clinical trials for the National Cholesterol Education Program Adult Treatment Panel III guidelines. Circulation 2004;110(2):227–39.

[120] Pearson TA, Blair SN, Daniels SR, et al. AHA guidelines for primary prevention of cardiovascular disease and stroke. 2002 update: consensus panel guide to comprehensive risk reduction for adult patients without coronary or other atherosclerotic vascular diseases. American Heart Association Science Advisory and Coordinating Committee. Circulation 2002;106:388–91.

[121] Padwal R, Majumdar SR, Johnson JA, et al. A systematic review of drug therapy to delay or prevent type 2 diabetes. Diabetes Care 2005;28:736–44.

[122] Clark LT. Improving compliance and increasing control of hypertension: needs of the special hypertensive populations. Am Heart J 1991;121:664–9.

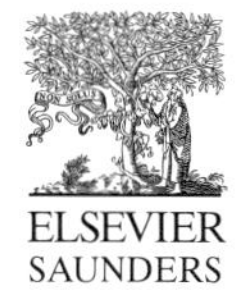

ELSEVIER
SAUNDERS

THE MEDICAL
CLINICS
OF NORTH AMERICA

Med Clin N Am 89 (2005) 1003–1031

Health Disparities in Transplantation: Focus on the Complexity and Challenge of Renal Transplantation in African Americans

Carlton J. Young, MD[a],*, Clifton Kew, MD[b]

[a]*Division of Transplantation, Department of Surgery, University of Alabama at Birmingham,
Lyons-Harrison Research Building, LHRB 728, 1530 3rd Avenue S,
Birmingham, AL 35294-0007, USA*
[b]*Division of Nephrology, Department of Medicine, University of Alabama at Birmingham,
Tinsley Harrison Tower, THT 643, 1530 3rd Avenue S,
Birmingham, AL 35294-0006, USA*

The year 2004 marked the 50th anniversary of the first successful renal transplant performed by Dr. Joseph Murray; subsequently, the field of renal transplantation has grown exponentially. A greater understanding of the immune system has resulted in the advent of numerous immunosuppressive agents. These immunosuppressive agents have lowered 1-year acute rejection rates to less than 10%, and 1-year graft survival rates for living- and deceased-donor renal allografts now routinely surpass 93%. In addition, long-term patient survival following transplantation has surpassed survival on dialysis for all ethnicities [1].

African Americans and whites have benefited from these advances; however, equivalent long-term success eludes African Americans who are also disadvantaged in gaining access to renal transplantation. Constituting approximately 38% of those waiting for a renal transplant, African Americans receive less than 28% of the deceased-donor renal allografts each year. These glaring discrepancies initiated an examination by the transplant community of the transplant process at several levels, including access to the transplant system, allocation of organs, and management after engraftment.

* Corresponding author.
E-mail address: cjyoung@uab.edu (C.J. Young).

This review summarizes the obstacles for African Americans to end-stage renal disease (ESRD) care, focusing on transplantation. Factors that predispose African Americans for ESRD, impede this ethnic group from timely transplantation, and negatively influence graft survival are examined. Possible solutions to these persistent problems are offered.

End-stage renal disease in African Americans

African Americans are significantly more likely to develop ESRD than whites [2–5] and constitute almost a third of those with ESRD [6]. Agodoa [7] observed that the earlier onset and more severe disease in racial and ethnic minority populations might be partly explained by lifestyle choices and impaired access to health care, compounded by lower socioeconomic status. The United States Renal Data System (USRDS) annual report from 2004 noted that African Americans in the United States have a disproportionately greater incidence and prevalence rates of ESRD (Fig. 1) [7]. The 2003 USRDS annual report noted that the overall adjusted incidence rate of ESRD was 334 per million for whites versus 998 per million for African Americans, which represents a quadrupling of the overall incidence of ESRD since 1980 when the USRDS first collected data to monitor the incidence and prevalence of chronic kidney disease (CKD) and ESRD in the United States [8].

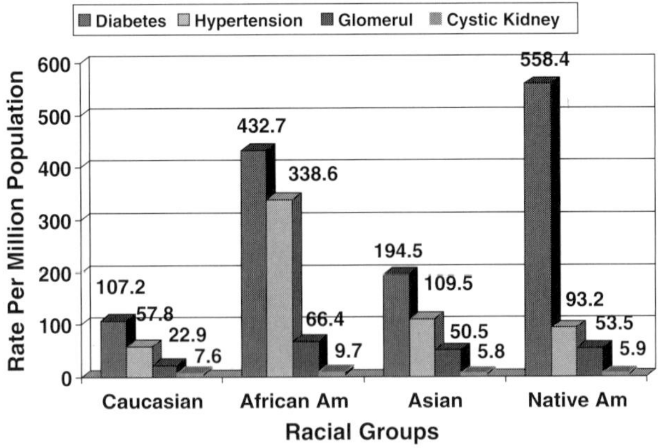

Fig. 1. Incidence rates of ESRD due to diabetes, hypertension, and other renal disease according to ethnicity. (*From* Agodoa L. Lessons from chronic renal diseases in African American Americans: treatment implications. Ethn Dis 2003;13:S120; with permission.)

Although some of the factors contributing to these alarming rates of ESRD among African Americans have been identified, the exact reasons why these disparities exist and continue have yet to be fully elucidated. For the time being, ESRD in the United States is likely to remain disproportionately higher in Americans of African descent [9] and, therefore, result in many more ethnic minority patients awaiting renal replacement therapy.

Approximately 70% of all new adult ESRD cases in the United States are due to hypertension and diabetes mellitus. Glomerulonephritis and cystic kidney diseases constitute about 10% of the cases (see Fig. 1) [7]. Regardless of the diagnosis, African Americans are at greater risk than whites of ultimately requiring dialysis or transplantation [6]. In the United States, diabetes is the leading cause of ESRD: the prevalence of diabetes in African-American men is nearly 50% greater than in white men, and African-American women are 100% more likely to have diabetes than whites [10].

Krop and colleagues [11] noted that African Americans with diabetes mellitus had early renal function decline three times that of whites. More than 80% of this disparity has been attributed to lower socioeconomic status, suboptimal health behaviors, and suboptimal control of blood glucose level and blood pressure. This trend is likely to continue because the incidence of type 2 diabetes mellitus is fueled by the increasing prevalence of obesity.

The second most common cause of ESRD is hypertension. The prevalence of hypertension among African Americans has increased substantially [12,13] and is the highest in the world [14]. Among young African Americans aged 20 to 44 years, the incidence of hypertension is 20 times that of whites [15]. In another study, the age-adjusted prevalence of hypertension in African Americans is 32.4%, which is nearly 40% higher than non-Hispanic whites (23.3%) and Mexican Americans (22.6%) [16]. Hypertension is a major contributing factor in the increased prevalence of ESRD seen in the African-American population, leading to dialysis or transplantation [17].

This pattern of hypertensive ESRD is unique among African Americans; it has remained a leading cause of ESRD for all ages—from the pediatric group (uncommon in other racial/ethnic groups) through the geriatric population [7]. The pilot phase of the African-American Study of Kidney Disease and Hypertension noted that 50% of renal biopsy samples taken from participants with the clinical diagnosis of hypertensive kidney disease histologically appeared exclusively as arterio- and arteriolonephrosclerosis [18,19]. Among several mechanistic theories that have been proposed is the possibility that environmental and genetic factors (excess salt intake superimposed on a genetic predisposition to salt retention) may lead to low-renin hypertension [9,20,21]. African Americans may have a predisposition to the deleterious effects of hypertension on renal function, even if blood pressures are well controlled [5,9,22]. Added to these physiologic variables are the socioeconomic and educational disadvantages often encountered by African Americans and other ethnic minorities, many of whom never received care for their hypertension before developing irreversible kidney failure [4,23–25]. In sum, there are proportionately more African Americans entering the ESRD network, yet as a group, they are significantly under-represented in the population receiving renal transplants.

Renal transplantation in African Amercians

Thirty years ago, dialysis was considered optimal treatment for patients with chronic renal failure [26]. Improved outcomes in renal transplantation challenged this assumption [3]. Renal transplantation reduces mortality, improves quality of life, and is less costly than dialysis [27–29]. The benefits of renal transplantation have been shown regardless of sex, race, age, or cause of ESRD [1]. It is unfortunate that access to this life-prolonging modality is not equivalent among all ethnicities: African-American ESRD patient access to transplantation is limited relative to whites [3]; African Americans are less than half as likely to receive a kidney transplant [6]; and the median waiting time for a cadaver kidney is twice as long (1185 versus 605 days) for an African-American candidate [30].

Barriers to transplant candidacy

In 2000, 96,192 patients (87%) were started on hemodialysis as their initial mode of therapy. African Americans represented 29% of that incident dialysis population, fewer than the 63% who were whites. Despite the lower incidence, proportionately more African Americans were in the prevalent dialysis population compared with whites (38% and 54%, respectively) [31]. Despite the hefty representation of African Americans on hemodialysis, the annual death rate was 181/1000 patient years, lower than the 284.7/1000 patient years for whites [31]. The lower rate has been attributed to African-American patients faring better than other ethnicities on dialysis; however, this conclusion may be incorrect. Because African Americans on hemodialysis tend to be younger, a possible explanation for this difference in death rate is that African Americans on dialysis are healthier than whites on dialysis and are better able to withstand dialysis treatment. In 2002, 54% of patients on dialysis under age 50 years were African Americans; this percentage decreased to 39% for those over age 50 years [31]. It follows that African-American patients who are suitable candidates for renal transplantation are not being transplanted but are waiting on dialysis. Conversely, the older, less healthy, and more likely untransplantable patients (ie, patients from ethnic majorities with multiple comorbidities) are dying on dialysis and possibly creating the false impression that death rates are higher. Between 1997 and 2000, 49,963 deceased-donor renal allografts were transplanted in the United States. Of these allografts, 35,532 (71%) were transplanted into whites, whereas 11,667 (23%) went to African Americans. Therefore, it was surmised that the decrease in the proportion of whites in the prevalent population was mainly due to their referral for renal transplantation and not patient death [7].

Debate continues as to whether there are discrepancies in the referral of African Americans compared with other ethnic groups. Thamer and colleagues [32] conducted a nationwide mail survey of United States nephrologists consisting of hypothetic patient scenarios, for which 53% of nephrologists responded. These investigators concluded that female sex and Asian ethnicity but not African-American ethnicity decreased the likelihood of recommendation or referral for renal transplantation. Soucie and colleagues [33] in an earlier study, however, found that African-American ESRD patients were less likely to be identified as transplant candidates than whites.

In another study to gauge sentiment among referring nephrologists, Ayanian and colleagues [34] conducted a survey of 278 nephrologists from four different regions in the United States. These physicians were asked to comment on the quality of life and survival of African-American and white patients undergoing renal transplantation and the reasons for racial differences in access to transplantation. To balance this survey, 606 of their patients were also interviewed.

Nephrologists were less likely to believe that transplantation improves survival for African Americans as much as whites (69% versus 81%, $P = .001$), even though they believed that it improves quality of life equally (84% versus 86%). When asked why they did not believe that African Americans were referred as often for transplantation, they cited patient preference (66%), availability of living donors (66%), failure to complete evaluations (53%), and comorbid conditions (52%). Few physicians believed that patient–physician communication and trust (38%) or physician bias (12%) were important factors. Conversely, African-American patients stated that they possessed a lack of information about the benefits of renal transplantation compared with their white counterparts (55% versus 74%, $P = .006$).

African-American physicians were more likely than white physicians to view patients' desire for transplantation as an important reason for racial differences in care, but the small number of African-American physicians yielded a wide confidence interval for this finding (odds ratio, 9.2; 95% confidence interval, 1.1–77.1; $P = .04$). African-American patients were also less likely to state that they received some or a lot of information about transplantation from their nephrologists (60% versus 72%, $P = .007$) when the nephrologists practiced in two or more dialysis facilities. It was concluded that nearly one third of the nephrologists did not perceive a survival benefit of renal transplantation over dialysis therapy for African-American patients, so they did not recommend this procedure as strongly to their African-American patients.

There is an apparent wide gap in communication among nephrologists and their African-American patients that is not widely recognized. Nephrologists were far more likely to believe that differences in referral rates among ethnicities were primarily due to patient preferences rather than from problems with communication, trust, or racial bias that may influence physician action or inaction. These observations differed sharply from studies that showed only small differences in patient preferences by race and showed larger racial differences in the quality of communication.

In another study, Ayanian and colleagues [35] found that African-American ESRD patients, after being fully informed of their options, preferred transplantation over dialysis as often as whites but were significantly less likely to proceed rapidly to transplantation [31]. They also noted that African Americans were less likely to appear on waiting lists or undergo transplantation due to associated factors (place of residence, educational level, functionality on dialysis, and associated medical comorbidity). Epstein and others [36] reiterated these discrepancies when they reviewed 1518 patient records among those who started dialysis in 1996/1997 from five states and the District of Columbia. These investigators found that African Americans were less likely than whites to be rated as appropriate candidates for transplantation and were more likely to have incomplete evaluations (46.5% versus 38.8%, $P < .001$). Of those patients deemed appropriate, African Americans were less likely to be referred for evaluation (90.1% versus 98%, $P = .008$), to be placed on the waiting list (71% versus 86.7%, $P = .007$), or to undergo transplantation (16.9% versus 52%, $P < .001$).

Other investigators found African Americans to be a third less likely than whites to appear on a transplant waiting list within the first year of Medicare eligibility [37]. This finding is troubling because Medicare mandates transplant evaluation for all dialysis patients. Moreover, the significantly lower rate of transplant activation in optimal African-American candidates is disturbing because young and healthy patients are likely to derive the greatest benefit (ie, longevity, quality of life) from transplantation compared with patients considered marginal because of advanced age or comorbid illness [38].

Compounding this problem is the evaluation process. At the University of Alabama at Birmingham (UAB), a referral initiates a two- to three-day inpatient evaluation that reduces the need for outpatient testing and results in 80% of evaluated whites and 76% of African Americans being proved acceptable transplant candidates [39]. This process may be unique to UAB; most other centers perform the majority of the evaluation as an outpatient. Transplant evaluation requires potential candidates to complete a complex array of interviews and medical screenings, a daunting outpatient task for many ESRD patients with limited resources. As a result, African Americans accounted for only 28% of new listings in 1997, and current data indicate that disparity in referral persists [30,40]. In 1998, Kasiske and colleagues [40] found that whites were more than twice as likely as African Americans to be wait-listed before dialysis.

Barriers to deceased-donor transplantation

After candidacy is established, African Americans are at a disadvantage in obtaining a deceased-donor transplant. The United Network for Organ Sharing (UNOS) allocation policy mandates ABO blood type identity. Although this is a necessary policy, African-American candidates, by nature of the donor pool (predominantly white), are disadvantaged by a pre-dilection for ABO blood types associated with longer waits [36]. Although dialysis is life prolonging, extended periods on dialysis are detrimental to subsequent renal allograft survival. Meier-Kriesche and colleagues [41] analyzed 73,103 primary adult renal transplants from the USRDS (1988–1997). Wait time on dialysis greater than 6 months resulted in a progressive increase in the relative risk for patient death following transplantation ($P < .001$). In addition, African-American transplant candidates are more likely to demonstrate significant anti–major histocompatibility complex (MHC) reactivity (presensitization) than comparable whites, which more often results in a positive crossmatch that precludes transplantation [37,42]. ESRD patients presensitized to 20% or more potential donors wait substantially longer for transplantation; an African-American patient receiving a deceased-donor transplant is 40% more likely than a white patient to have met this criterion [30].

Another important facet in receiving a renal allograft is the relative weight of MHC matching in the former UNOS allocation algorithm (Table 1). Wait-listed transplant candidates accumulate "points." When a kidney becomes available, the medically suitable candidate with the most points is designated to receive the organ. Based on the assumption that similarity in MHC antigen expression (ie, matching) between donor and recipient optimizes outcomes, matching was the predominant variable determining allocation of deceased-donor kidneys [43].

The primary benefit of this allocation algorithm was unintentionally conferred on the predominantly white recipients of completely matched grafts, with marginal impact on outcomes across other match grades, especially among African-American recipients. This trend was recognized over a decade ago with few inter-racial transplants occurring with greater than three (of six) matched MHC alleles [44,45]. At UAB, only 1 of 33 fully matched cadaver kidneys went to a black recipient [46]. Takemoto and colleagues [47] reviewed the UNOS database from 1987 to September 1999 to determine the efficacy of sharing HLA matched kidneys. Although they showed a great benefit to this sharing, African Americans received only 8% of the 7614 matched kidneys. Conversely, 30% of mismatched kidneys went

Table 1
Former renal allocation point system for allocating cadaver kidneys in the United States

Criterion	Points awarded
Zero antigen mismatch	Mandatory share
MHC mismatches	
0 BDR	7
1 BDR	5
2 BDR	2
Presensitization	
Panel reactive antibody $\geq 80\%$	4
Waiting time	
Longest wait (then fractional)	1
Each year on list	1
Age	
<11 y	4
11–18 y	3

Data from United Network for Organ Sharing. Point change results from UNOS study. UNOS Update 1994;Dec:18.

to African-American recipients, approximating the frequency with which African Americans appear on the waiting list [48,49]. Even the proponents of the former allocation system conceded that racial disparity existed [50,51]. This fact was made more unacceptable when improved immuno-suppressive medications reduced the impact of matching on allograft survival [48,51–54]. The core of the former point system was implemented in the 1980s when demonstrable incremental benefit of improved HLA compatibility between donor and recipient was evident. Now, at least two groups of investigators estimate that the overall national impact of optimal HLA matching is relatively small, improving graft survival by only 1%–2% [55,56]. In addition, early reports documented no statistical benefit of matching among African Americans, a finding attributed to the difficulty of obtaining enough good matches in this population for meaningful analysis [50,51]. Current data indicate a benefit for African Americans of 5%–6% (in graft survival at 3 years) in the few patients able to receive completely matched grafts, and improvement in allograft half-life from 5.4 to 8.4 years (the latter still being $<$ 9.7 years expected for white recipients of mismatched kidneys) [48,49].

A new UNOS renal allocation scheme was implemented in May 2003 to address discrepancies in kidney allocation that result from a heterogeneous HLA donor and recipient population (Table 2). This new scheme has been an important step in rectifying the allocation of renal allografts. Inasmuch as the former UNOS algorithm perpetuated ethnic disparities, major changes have occurred while preserving mandatory sharing of phenotypi-cally identical (completely matched) kidneys because it improves transplant outcomes and, despite identifiable adverse impact on access for African Americans, removes relatively few organs from the overall pool [48,57,58].

Table 2
United Network for Organ Sharing kidney allocation

Criterion	Points awarded
Zero antigen mismatch	Mandatory share
MHC mismatches	
0 BDR	2
1 BDR	1
2 BDR	0
Presensitization	
Panel reactive antibody $\geq 80\%$	4
Waiting time	
Longest wait (then fractional)	1
Each year on list	1
Age	
< 11 y	4
11–18 y	3

Implemented May 2003.

Beyond phenotypic identity, allocation of points for "partial" matching was determined indefensible. A 1995 analysis confirmed that "matching points" were accumulated disproportionately by whites and awarded for match quality that produced outcomes no better (two mismatches) or worse (three mismatches) than the national average [41].

In response, the algorithm was modified to its current form; the impact of these modifications on minority access is being assessed [59]. A recent regional study involving the New England Organ Bank documented that elimination of points for partial matching indeed improved access for minorities without compromising outcomes [60]. Other modifications are possible. Currently, UNOS allows local variances based on the concept of "acceptable mismatches" that, at least theoretically, preserve the benefits of matching while offering more equitable allocation [50]. Although some remain unenthusiastic about the potential benefit of such an approach, prospective evaluation of its merits is pending [49]. Alternatively, in light of increasing recognition of the influence of nonimmunologic factors (particularly early graft function and donor age) on long-term survival, it may be time to formulate a completely new paradigm for organ allocation [61–63].

Barriers to living donation

Not only are African Americans significantly less likely to identify a deceased donor, they also have more difficultly in locating a potential live donor [39,64]. The advantages of live donation are the possible avoidance of dialysis, shorter waiting times, and improved graft survival over deceased-donor transplantation. At UAB, 1-year deceased-donor graft survival is 93% for African Americans and whites, whereas living donor 1-year graft survival is 97% for both. Potential African-American donors, however, were more likely to be excluded because of a previously undiagnosed comorbidity [39]. At UAB, only 13% of acceptable African-American transplant candidates (versus 33% of whites) ultimately received a kidney from a living donor. This percentage reflects a national trend [30,65]. Although better education and surgical advances (eg, laparoscopic nephrectomy) have increase the overall numbers of live donors, factors such as pre-existing comorbidity in family members may limit their impact among African-American ESRD patients [64,66]. With fewer live donors available, African-American transplant candidates are more dependent on the deceased-donor kidney supply and do not receive the advantages of living donor transplantation to the same extent as whites [30,55,57].

Outcomes in African Americans after renal transplantation

African-American recipients of renal allografts fare substantially worse with long-term graft survival compared with whites and other minorities [6,30,52,67–70]. Renal allograft half-life for African Americans is only 30%–40% that of whites [69,71,72]. For reasons heretofore unexplained, decreasing rates of early rejection coupled with improved 1-year graft survival, which is similar among ethnicities, has not translated into improved long-term graft survival for African Americans [51,68,70,71]. For example, over the last several years, 1-year graft survival rates for African Americans at UAB have been more than 90%; however, by 3 years, a trend toward increasing graft loss was seen (Figs. 2 and 3). There is no single answer for this conundrum. A multiplicity of factors, ranging from socioeconomic status to physiology, affects African Americans negatively,

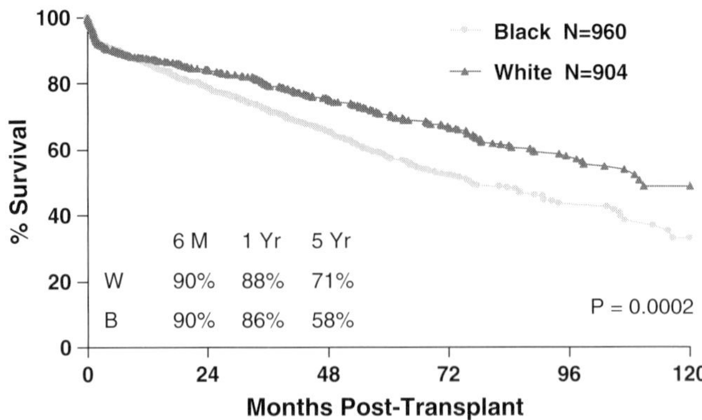

Fig. 2. Deceased-donor graft survival by ethnicity, 1991–2001. B, black; M, month; W, white; Yr, year.

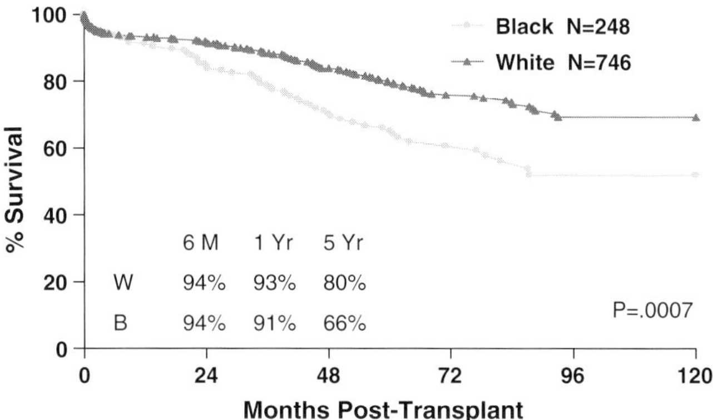

Fig. 3. Living donor graft survival by ethnicity, 1991–2001. B, black; M, month; W, white; Yr, year.

making renal allograft survival more tenuous. In an effort to corral this problem, potential impacting variables can be divided into nonimmunologic and immunologic factors.

Nonimmunologic factors

Hypertension

Poor renal allograft survival is associated with worsening hypertension. It has been shown that allograft recipients with blood pressures greater than 140/90 mm Hg at 1 year have worse allograft survival than those with blood pressures less than 140/90 mm Hg [73]. As previously stated, African Americans are significantly more likely to suffer from hypertension than whites. Poorly controlled post-transplant hypertension has been shown to be more detrimental toward renal graft survival in African-American recipients than in whites [74]. This problem tends to be exacerbated after transplantation through the use of immunosuppressive medications that raise blood pressure in 60%–80% of patients [75]. Calcinurin inhibitors (cyclosporine and tacrolimus) are mainstays of immunosuppressive therapy but cause hypertension by worsening systemic vasoconstriction. Some believe that renovascular hypertension is also a consequence, which in turn causes decreased glomerular filtration and enhanced sodium retention [76].

Corticosteroids increase blood pressure through sodium retention and increased plasma volume [77]. These mechanisms of action may have greater impact on African Americans because hypertension in African Americans may be associated with abnormal sodium metabolism (ie, reduced ability to excrete salt), leading to low-renin hypertension and variability among ethnicities in the endothelin-1 system [8,20,21,78–80]. Recently, the standard at which a patient is deemed hypertensive was adjusted from 140/90 mm Hg to 130/80 mm Hg. The previous standard, however, was set in the white population. Some investigators are now suggesting that this target may not be adequate for all ethnic groups. In response, a national task force suggests that African Americans with renal dysfunction be treated to a lower blood pressure [81].

Controversy also exists regarding the best antihypertensive medications for African Americans in the nontransplant population. These questions are being addressed in the ongoing African-American Study of Kidney Disease and Hypertension clinical trial [82]. Current data, however, indicate that in the presence of proteinuria (300 mg/24 hours), disease progression is more rapid unless angiotensin-converting enzyme inhibitors are used [83–85]. Therefore, assuming that there would be similar effects in the transplant population, this modality, while being investigated, should be offered to all patients who might benefit. In the authors' clinical practice, angiotensin-converting enzyme inhibitors are used extensively in allograft recipients for hypertensive control, specifically when an allograft recipient develops proteinuria. These findings mandate that blood pressure control in African Americans be given the same weight as maintaining adequate levels of immunosuppressive medications. Although daunting, aggressive management by transplant physicians and community physicians can have a positive impact on long-term renal allograft function in African-American recipients.

Socioeconomic status and noncompliance

These two entities play a significant role in allograft survival because lower income levels have been associated with increased risk of late graft loss [86]. Of all the factors noted to impact graft survival in African Americans, socioeconomic status remains the least clearly defined. The long history of social and economic repression in the United States has created a significant gap between most African Americans and the general population. Although a significant number of the poorer members of the majority population including whites are clearly present in all parts of the United States, the number of African Americans with incomes below the federal poverty level is fourfold greater than the number of whites at this level [87]. As a result, African Americans are much more likely to be dependent on public assistance programs such as Medicare and Medicaid for health insurance and medication coverage.

Noncompliance, as a function of socioeconomic status, has been shown to be a significant predictor of graft loss for African Americans and for whites [88–90]. Didlake and colleagues [91] noted that compliance was a significant factor in late allograft loss, and Gaston and coworkers [92] found that 77% of recipients with chronic rejection were noncompliant. Moreover, a study by Kalil and colleagues [93] noted that graft survival was negatively associated with patients on medical assistance compared with those with adequate income.

Butkus and coworkers [94] examined the impact of poverty and other socioeconomic factors on graft survival. They took detailed histories of 450 consecutive candidates (128 who underwent transplantation: 89 African American, 39 white). Variables examined included household income, literacy, marital status, insurance coverage, years of education, pretransplant compliance, history of substance abuse, and pre- and post-transplant demographics. Median household income of African Americans was significantly lower compared with whites, and a greater percentage of African Americans were below the federal poverty level (58% versus 31%, $P < .005$). More whites had private insurance (44% versus 16%, $P < .05$), whereas African Americans were predominately covered by Medicaid (65%), alone (8%) or with Medicare (57%). An equal percentage of African Americans and whites were covered with Medicare alone (19% versus 22%). Eleven percent of African Americans and 3% of whites had a pretransplant history of noncompliance, and 10% of African Americans and 3% of whites had post-transplant noncompliance, but these differences were not significant. One-year patient and graft survival was not different between African Americans and whites, but African Americans were twice as likely to experience an acute rejection episode (34.8% versus 19.4%, $P < .05$) or have an immunologic cause of their graft loss. Allograft loss, when analyzed by the proportional-hazards model, was significantly more likely to occur in African Americans whose income was below the federal poverty level. This finding was closely coupled with a pretransplant history of substance abuse or a post-transplant history of noncompliance but was not related to pretransplant noncompliance.

Isaacs and colleagues [95] examined the UNOS registry of 14,617 living related–donor renal transplants from January 1, 1988 to December 31, 1994. African Americans were 1.8 times as likely as whites to lose their grafts at 8 years despite adjusting for confounding variables; 2031 patients lost their grafts at 8 years, with most of the losses due to chronic rejection. African Americans were more likely than other ethnicities to lose their grafts due to chronic rejection. In contradistinction to the prior studies that showed a significant impact of noncompliance in African Americans leading to graft failure, Isaacs and colleagues [95] noted that although the noncompliance rate for African Americans (5.4%) was higher than for whites (3.7%), this difference could not account for the racial differences in outcomes. It is interesting that Asians had the highest rate of noncompliance (15.4%) but had the lowest rate of acute rejection (11.5%) compared with African Americans (24.2%) and whites (22.5%).

When loss of Medicare benefits for immunosuppressive drugs forced discontinuation of cyclosporine in a cohort of impoverished patients, only the African-American recipients suffered adverse consequences of rejection and graft loss [96]. Subsequently, when similarly disadvantaged patients received cyclosporine by way of an indigent care program, demonstrable adverse outcomes evaporated among black recipients [97]. An analysis of

USRDS data revealed that extension of Medicare immunosuppressant coverage from 1 to 3 years after transplantation exerted its greatest relative benefit among those in the lower socioeconomic strata [86]. It is likely that further extension of Medicare immunosuppressive drug benefits beyond 3 years would provide a beneficial impact [98].

The difference in graft survival among ethnicities as a factor of insurance coverage was examined when Oliver and coworkers [99] looked at African-American military personnel who received renal transplants. This group of recipients had the same access to health care as whites. These investigators found that when health care access was equivalent, regardless of socioeconomic status, no racial differences in graft survival were detected.

Limiting these investigations is the ability to accurately determine noncompliance rates. It is very difficult to capture all noncompliant episodes. It is safe to say that noncompliance in the African-American patient is more likely to lead to graft loss compared with other ethnicities. This fact indirectly points to physiologic differences between African Americans and other ethnicities that make them less likely to tolerate lapses in immunosuppressive medications, which may be related to hyperimmune responsiveness, as discussed in the following section.

Drug absorption

Absorption of immunosuppressive medications has been identified as one of the most important factors in determining outcome following renal transplantation. Immunosuppressive medication effectiveness is concentration dependent, requires close blood level monitoring, and is a mainstay of follow-up care. As the field of transplantation evolved, it became apparent that some medications were more poorly absorbed in certain formulations. For example, the original formulation of cyclosporine was noted to have an extremely variably absorption profile. In 1995, a new microemulsion formulation significantly improved bioavailability.

Concomitant with this revelation, investigators began to question whether ethnic differences existed to explain differences in outcomes and acute rejection episodes. Pharmacokinetic variances in African Americans for cyclosporine have been noted. Circadian variations in African Americans have been postulated as a reason for high early-morning cyclosporine levels and subtherapeutic daytime levels [100]. When dosing is based on trough levels, the dose of cyclosporine could be lowered inappropriately, leading to an increased risk of rejection. Diurnal measurements have been suggested but are logistically unreasonable; however, measuring C_2, the cyclosporine levels 2 hours after dosing was found to correlate best with drug exposure among whites [101,102].

Neylan [102] examined the efficacy of tacrolimus versus cyclosporine among African Americans and whites in a multicenter trial and concluded that tacrolimus was more effective than cyclosporine in preventing acute rejection in African-American and white patients. It is interesting that African-American patients required a 37% mean higher dose of tacrolimus than whites to achieve comparable blood concentrations. This finding was similar to that reported by Andrews and colleagues [103] who found that the mean dose of tacrolimus for African-American patients was 96% higher than for white patients. Heifets and coworkers [104] noted that African Americans had significantly higher clearance of the drug and a significantly lower area under the curve.

The absorption and the clearance of tacrolimus are dependent on intestinal P-glycoprotein (the product of the multiple drug resistance gene MDR-1) and cytochrome P450 (CYP3A-gene), respectively. Variability exists among ethnic populations, making dose adjustments necessary to achieve adequate levels to prevent rejection [102]. Macphee and colleagues [105] found that a single nucleotide polymorphism in one of the CYP3A genes that codes for hepatic cytochrome P450 was strongly associated with activity that resulted in more efficient metabolism of orally absorbed tacrolimus. This allelic modification was more common in African Americans. In addition, intestinal P-glycoprotein polymorphism was noted to be variable among ethnicities. Macphee and colleagues [105] concluded that the major absorption pathway in African Americans was less effective than in whites and that the elimination pathway in the liver by way of the cytochrome P450 enzyme was more efficient. After dosing with tacrolimus, levels were 50% lower in African Americans with the same dosing regimen. In turn, tacrolimus dose requirements were higher in patients expressing this substitution. It is interesting that African-American and white patients who did not have this substitution had the same dose requirements. These researchers concluded that the CYP3AP1 genotype is a more important factor than ethnicity in determining tacrolimus pharmacokinetics. A lesser association was noted with MDR-1 polymorphism.

Collectively, these observations may partially explain lower tacrolimus and cyclosporine levels in African Americans who are more likely than whites to express these polymorphisms. To achieve comparable levels in African-American patients, higher doses are required. Identification of such patients is essential to anticipate the higher dosing requirements needed to compensate for the increased activity of the gene [106,107]. Even though additional studies are needed to confirm these findings, they are intriguing as a possible reason why rejection rates are higher and graft survival is lower in African Americans than in whites.

Immunologic factors

African Americans are disadvantaged because of immunologic factors that may be exacerbated by the nonimmunologic factors heretofore discussed. In an era in which similarities rather than differences among peoples are advocated, acknowledgment of these ethnic differences may hold the key to why there is such variation in graft survival for African Americans compared with other ethnicities.

Major histocompatibility complex polymorphism

African Americans are more likely to exhibit MHC polymorphism that, in turn, may lead to inferior graft survival [108]. This plieomorphic diversity, compared with a more homogeneous white population, has made matching more difficult because most deceased-donor kidneys are white. Moreover, African Americans are more likely to have uncharacterized HLA alleles that make matching more complicated. With the advent of newer histocompatibility techniques, more of these alleles are being identified, but the existence of this greater diversity indirectly implicates genetic differences as a possible reason for an observed heightened immune response.

Sensitization

African Americans demonstrate a greater propensity to exhibit presensitization to MHC antigens [51,70] that leads to a heightened immune response following transplantation. Moreover, presensitization makes it more difficult to find a suitable kidney for an African-American recipient because the likelihood of preformed antibodies is greater, resulting in a positive crossmatch. Compared with other ethnicities, African Americans have a more vigorous response to blood transfusions and other sources of antigen exposure. This heightened immune response is thought to be directly responsible for poorer graft survival. This idea is not surprising because it is known that graft loss, primarily acute rejection, is a T-cell mediated phenomenon. In addition, chronic allograft nephropathy may also have a strong immunologic component.

Matching

Controversy exists over whether better matching (and presumed lower acute rejection rates) truly leads to improved graft survival among African-American recipients [40,51,109]. HLA mismatches of one to six alleles have about a 10% difference in graft survival, even for African Americans [110]. This observation augmented the decision to revise the UNOS renal allocation scheme. The A locus had been removed previously, but a fierce debate raged as to the efficacy of removing the B locus.

The fact that African-American patients waited significantly longer for a renal transplant prompted the implementation of a new allocation scheme that eliminated points for the HLA-B locus on May 7, 2003. Port and colleagues [111] compared the effects of allocation before and after the change. The study population consisted of 8254 patients who received a solitary donor transplant from September 7, 2002 to September 6, 2003. Of these, 2758 (33%) received their transplant after the policy change. Nonwhite recipients experienced a 7.2% increase in access to renal allografts (36% prepolicy change, 38.6% postpolicy change). Similar increases in access were seen for pediatric, mismatched antigen, and highly sensitized patients. One concern was that there were fewer zero-mismatched or perfectly matched grafts that were transplanted.

Rebellato and coworkers [112] expressed concern that removing the B locus in addition to the prior removal of the A locus would increase the rate of graft loss, leading to the sensitization of African-American recipients and a decrease in their ability to receive a future transplant. They cited a significant difference in graft survival between 0,1,2 MHC loci B and DR mismatching and 3,4 MHC loci B and DR mismatching ($P = .0022$) despite a 69% use of induction therapy. It is too early to evaluate the impact of the policy change on graft loss and the subsequent sensitization of African-American recipients on future transplant candidacy. For now, the change in the allocation scheme has, at least in part, achieved what it intended: improve access for a disadvantaged population with greater MHC polymorphism.

Lastly and more disturbing, living-donor kidneys with genotypically identical, nonpolymorphous one- and two-haplotype matches fare significantly worse in African Americans than in whites [66,90]. Of all the HLA combinations available, one would surmise that a perfectly matched living-donor kidney should overcome the immunologic effects suspected in causing poor graft survival. This is not the case for African Americans and clearly implicates other confounding variables outside of HLA matching as possible causes for increased graft loss.

Hyperimmune responsiveness/cytokine polymorphism

Fundamental to T-cell proliferation and clonal expansion is the role of cytokines. These molecules play a crucial role in the trafficking and regulation of the immune response. The T-helper cell 1 (Th1) cytokines—interleukin (IL)-2, tumor necrosis factor α, and interferon (IFN)-γ—have been implicated as being the main cytokines involved in cell-mediated immunity. Of these, IL-2 has been the most prominent because two of the major immunosuppressive agents (the calcinurin inhibitors) target the production of this molecule. In contrast, the Th2 cytokines, IL-4 and IL-10, have been shown to be involved in the control of humoral responses and have been implicated in allograft protection [113,114]. Lastly, the Th3 type cytokines, of which transforming growth factor (TGF)-β is prominent, have been associated with allograft outcome depending on the interaction between Th1 and Th2 cytokines [114]. Cytokine production has been suggested to be under genetic control [115].

The binding of T cells to antigen-presenting cells (APCs) is mediated through adhesion molecules, including intercellular adhesion molecule 1, vascular adhesion molecule 1, and leukocyte function–associated antigen 1, which are partly induced by surgical trauma [116]. Ischemia/reperfusion injury accentuates an environment that promotes the upregulation of MHC class II antigens that eventually facilitates a cascade of signals (initiated by the release of cytokines) that drive the immune response [117,118]. As such, it reasonable to surmise that if MHC polymorphism exists with an effect on outcomes in African Americans, then the same type of polymorphism in cytokines may result in a similar effect. It has been shown that allelic differences in pro- and anti-inflammatory cytokines might play a role in allograft survival and that developing a genetic cytokine profile might be useful in determining a patient's risk of rejection and subsequent modulation of their immunosuppressive medications [119–124].

Cytokine polymorphisms are usually the result of single nucleotide polymorphisms or di-nucleotide polymorphisms. For example, IL-2 has T→G substitution at position −330 relative to the transcription start site, which produces two alleles that have variable frequency within the population [125,126]. A clinical effect of this substitution (ie, relative IL-2 production levels), however, has not been documented [126]. McDaniel and colleagues [127] noted that cytokine gene polymorphism and gene expression levels were elevated in a group of African-American patients who had undergone renal transplantation. They measured cytokine genotypes and mRNA transcript levels of IL-2, TNF-α, TGF-β, IL-10, IL-6, and IFN-γ from peripheral blood cells. The high IL-2, high TGF-β, intermediate IFN-γ, and low IL-10 producing genotypes were associated with allograft rejection, whereas the low IFN-γ and high IL-10 producing genotypes were associated with protection of the renal allograft.

A heightened APC response might play a role in augmenting the immune responsiveness of African Americans who have significant cytokine polymorphism, much like MHC polymorphism plays a role in the enhancement of immune responses. After antigens are processed by APCs and expressed on their surfaces, costimulatory molecules are upregulated to aid in the cascade that drives the immune proliferation of lymphocytes. Hutchings and colleagues [128] found that African Americans were much more likely to express higher levels of costimulatory molecules than whites. They examined the surface antigen expression of peripheral blood mononuclear cells from African-American and white transplant patients by flow cytometry. These investigators noted that APCs from African Americans expressed higher levels of the B-7 costimulatory molecules CD80 and CD86 than APCs from whites over an extended period of time (120 months post-transplant) that are essential to T-cell allorecognition and proliferation. Moreover, CD80 expression from African Americans was consistently increased compared with whites even when white patients began to have a diminution in their CD80 expression.

A more aggressive mixed lymphocyte response was also seen in African Americans as demonstrated by significantly more lymphocyte proliferation. When B7 and its counter-receptors CD28 and CD152 (CTLA-4) are blocked, rejection can be prevented and tolerance induced in experimental models [129,130]. Hutchings and colleagues [127] concluded that the proportion of APCs from African Americans was significantly higher than from whites and that these cells expressed high levels of the B7 costimulatory molecules CD80 and CD86. In addition, African-American patients required more immunosuppression to overcome this hyperimmune response and were less likely to develop donor-specific hyporesponsiveness over time.

Clinically, acute rejection is more common in African Americans. This observation has been partially associated with immunologic hyper-responsiveness [42,131]. Accordingly, many transplant clinicians have responded by treating their African-American patients with more intense immunosuppression [70,71,132]. These efforts have yet to improve significantly long-term graft survival despite a benefit in the short-term. These findings, although far from definitive, are intriguing because they strongly suggest that cytokine production has a direct bearing on the immunologic cascade and subsequent immune response. Further investigations are under way to define and characterize the complex interactions of these cytokines. Nevertheless, with more information, it might be possible to profile a patient and determine his or her likelihood of rejection.

Immunosuppression

The advancement of the transplantation could not have occurred without the development of effective immunosuppressive medications. Azathioprine and steroids were the foundation of immunosuppressive therapy until the introduction of cyclosporine in 1983. We now have a pharmacopeia of drugs with variable mechanisms of actions. New drugs have paralleled our understanding of immune system complexity. In 1995, mycophenolate mofetil, an inosine monophosphate dehydrogenase inhibitor that inhibits de novo guanine synthesis, supplanted azathioprine after lowering global acute rates from about 40% to 20%. Mycophenolate mofetil has become an essential part of triple-maintenance immunosuppression consisting of a calcinurin inhibitor and steroids with or without antibody induction therapy.

Meier-Kriesche and coworkers [133] reviewed all African-American and white adult renal transplant recipients (57,926 patients) in the USRDS who received a transplant between 1988 and 1998. Three-year death-censored graft survival for African Americans was 85.8% versus 75.1% ($P < .001$) for mycophenolate mofetil versus azathioprine. Conversely, white recipients had 3-year death-censored graft survival rates of 90.1% versus 86.4%, respectively ($P < .001$). During this time, acute rejection rates within 6 months of transplantation fell from 32.8% to 20.5% for African Americans and from 25.3% to 15.3% for whites. Collectively, mycophenolate mofetil had a significant impact on the risk of mortality and death-censored graft loss for both ethnic groups, but graft survival rates for African Americans still lagged behind. The introduction of mycophenolate mofetil strongly intimated the belief that African Americans needed more immunosuppression. The improved graft survival rates compared with azathioprine fueled the search for additional agents.

Over the last several years, sirolimus, a lymphocyte cell–cycle and vascular smooth muscle inhibitor, has been used more extensively in clinical trials. Hricik and colleagues [134] substituted sirolimus for mycophenolate mofetil in a regimen also consisting of tacrolimus and corticosteroids. Fifty-six African-American patients were enrolled in the study. The acute rejection rate within the first 3 months post transplant was no different between African Americans and whites. Moreover, actuarial 2-year patient survival, graft survival, and rejection-free graft survival was equivalent between the two groups.

In 1992, Gaston and coworkers [71] observed that African Americans required more immunosuppression to improve outcomes. More than a decade of transplantation has proved this observation correct. Many new and more potent immunosuppressive agents have arisen to significantly improve graft survival and decrease acute rejection rates in African Americans and in whites. Philosophic division persists as to the use of induction therapy and monoclonal and polyclonal antibodies. Some centers use some form of induction for all patients, whereas others use it selectively for high-risk patients (eg, delayed graft function, African Americans, repeat transplants, or those with high panel reactive antibody).

African Americans are not the same as whites immunologically, at least after receiving a renal allograft. These differences, though at times vexing, have shed great light on transplantation biology and fueled the search for more effective immunosuppressants. It is hoped that new combinations of current immunosuppressive medications, along with therapies heretofore undiscovered, may one day overcome the immunologic differences between African Americans and whites to improve long-term graft survival for everyone.

Conclusions and possible remedies to reduce health disparities in renal transplantation

The discrepancy between African Americans and whites with respect to treatment of ESRD is multifaceted and occurs at several stages of the transplant process. First, comorbid conditions such as diabetes and hypertension tend to affect African Americans at a higher rate and promote kidney disease. The rate at which African Americans develop CKD and ultimately reach ESRD will not change unless African Americans take charge of their health by assiduously adopting healthy lifestyles and daily living habits that are likely to ameliorate the tendency toward obesity, diabetes, and hypertension. Second, the cognitive processes and attitudes of health care providers need to change to facilitate the early and expeditious referral of African Americans and other minorities to dialysis and ultimately transplantation. Third, methods to simplify or "streamline" an outpatient pretransplant evaluation process may promote more equitable access to transplant candidacy. Fourth, timelier referral of African Americans for transplantation and better education of potential living donors and recipients are also likely to be of substantial benefit.

Effective communication is essential if these barriers to transplantation are to be overcome. Nephrologists and dialysis center staff can more effectively benefit patients by improving their ability to be more culturally sensitive. It is unfortunate that preconceived ideas of potential mistreatment and mistrust of the health care system remain present in the African-American community. Many of these perceptions have been entrenched since slavery when slaves were routinely denied access to the best medical care. More recent injustices such as the Tuskegee experiment still resonate with many African-American patients who continue to perceive the health care system as biased, unjust, and unequal. Klassen and colleagues [135] theorized that patients who experience a greater exposure to perceived discrimination are reluctant to risk new treatment options such as transplantation. Moreover, they have a lower expectation of successful outcome and are more likely to believe nothing can improve their chances.

Garg and colleagues [38] noted that African Americans are less likely than whites to participate in their medical decision making (particularly when treated by a white physician) and showed large differences in the extent to which African-American and white patients trust their physicians [35,136]. It is distressing that studies have indicated that some physicians make different treatment recommendations for their African-American and white patients [137]. The real and perceived differences in the level and quality of care are not lost on many minority patients who recognize these inconsistencies, which in turn increase their level of distrust for the medical community. These misconceptions can and must be reversed if access to transplantation is to achieve equality among all ethnicities. The specter of health disparities represents an egregious failure of the medical community in the United States. All efforts should be made to extend the potential of transplantation to everyone seeking ESRD, especially if they are free of comorbidities that preclude transplantation. This care should be provided regardless of the patient's ethnic background.

The problems associated with ABO blood types, matching, and presensitization are likely to prove more daunting. UNOS is committed to providing an equitable framework whereby all ethnicities are treated fairly, which is evidenced by the new renal allocation scheme. Although eliminating the donor shortage would obviously remedy any ethnic disparities in the allocation process, there is no indication of an impending deluge of donated organs. More African-American donors might theoretically provide more well-matched kidneys for African-American transplant candidates [51,138]; however, given the prevalence of ESRD and MHC polymorphisms among African Americans, this approach seems unlikely to resolve the donor issue [57,139]. Indeed, thanks to ongoing efforts to promote minority donation, the percentage of African-American donors now corresponds to black representation in the general population [140].

Nonimmune factors that effect transplant outcomes fall into two areas, those that are physical and those that are socioeconomic. Medical conditions such as diabetes and hypertension that can affect allograft longevity are present more often in African Americans than in whites. In addition, it appears that African Americans absorb immunosuppressant medications differently. Transplant physicians need to be aware of theses physical differences and adjust therapy appropriately. Addressing the socioeconomic differences is more pressing and more difficult. Affording immunosuppressant medications is a challenge for patients who are socioeconomically disadvantaged (many who are disproportionately African American). Currently, Medicare coverage lasts for 36 months, which is an improvement from 12 months, but many physicians have advocated for lifetime coverage so as not to foster economic noncompliance. African Americans suffer disproportionately because they are less tolerant of immunosuppression withdrawal than whites [96,141,142]. This loss of coverage has affected African Americans to a greater extent because a greater proportion is dependent on Medicare. As such, socioeconomically disadvantaged African Americans fair substantially worse. This nonimmunologic factor most likely potentiates the loss of renal allografts in African Americans. The situation is made worse because a return to dialysis is not only more costly than maintenance immunosuppression ($\sim$$5,000–$10,000/y versus $50,000/y) but survival of these patients is also significantly less than for patients with a functioning allograft. USRDS data indicate that the advantages of transplantation over dialysis, including significant prolongation of life expectancy, extend across ethnic boundaries [29].

Some changes have occurred already but they are limited. The federal government has made provisions to supply immunosuppressive medications for the life of some transplant recipients. Patients who are disabled, Medicare eligible, and over the age of 65 years are covered. Although this change is a step forward, global coverage is needed to ensure that noncompliance is not promoted due to socioeconomic hardship.

Despite the problems with access, the advent of newer immunosuppressive medications has resulted in negligible 1-year graft survival differences between African Americans and whites [30,74,90]. It is unfortunate, however, that beyond 2 years post transplant, the slope of graft loss for African Americans is steeper compared with whites. This discrepancy is highlighted by the observations of Koyama and colleagues [143] who found that for recipients of zero HLA-A, -B mismatched donor kidneys, African Americans had a renal allograft half-life of 8 years compared with 17 years for whites.

The interaction of immunologic and nonimmunologic factors affecting outcomes in African Americans receiving a renal allograft is substantial. Perhaps no other ethnic minority is influenced as much as this population. Of all the factors discussed, it appears that post-transplant hypertension, hyperimmune responsiveness, and socioeconomic status (as it relates to insurance coverage), exert the most influence on allograft survival.

Transplantation medicine is a microcosm of society. In no other discipline of medicine are issues of race, ethnicity, and equivalence so acutely discussed and acted upon. Through the continued efforts of dedicated clinicians and scientists, the conundrum of immunologic and nonimmunologic factors affecting graft survival in African Americans can be solved.

References

[1] Wolf RA, Ashby AV, Milford EI, et al. Comparison of mortality in all patients on dialysis, patients on dialysis awaiting transplantation, and recipients of a first cadaveric transplant. New Engl J Med 1999;341:725–32.

[2] Opelz G, Mickey MR, Terasaki PI. Influence of race on kidney transplant survival. Transplant Proc 1977;9:137–42.

[3] Eggers PW. Effect of transplantation on the Medicare end stage renal disease program. New Engl J Med 1988;318:223–9.

[4] Qualheim RE, Rostand SG, Kirk KA, et al. Changing patterns of end stage renal disease due to hypertension. Am J Kidney Dis 1991;18:336–43.

[5] Rostand SG. US minority groups and end-stage renal disease: a disproportionate share. Am J Kidney Dis 1992;19:411–3.

[6] United States Renal Data System. Excerpts from the USRDS 1999 annual data report. Am J Kidney Dis 1999;34(Suppl 1):S1–176.

[7] Agodoa L. Lessons from chronic renal diseases in African American Americans: treatment implications. Ethn Dis 2003;13(Suppl 2):118–24.

[8] US Renal Data System. USRDS 2003 annual data report: atlas of end-stage renal disease in the United States. Bethesda (MD): National Institutes of Health, National Institute of Diabetes and Digestive and Kidney Diseases; 2003.

[9] Hall WD, Kusek JW, Kirk KA, et al. Short-term effects of blood pressure control and antihypertensive drug regimen on glomerular filtration rate: the African-American Study of Kidney Disease and Hypertension Pilot Study. Am J Kidney Dis 1997;29:720–8.

[10] Crook ED, Harris J, Oliver B, et al. End-stage renal disease owing to diabetic nephropathy in Mississippi: an examination of factors influencing renal survival in a population prone to late referral. J Invest Med 2001;49(3):284–91.

[11] Krop JS, Coresh J, Chamblers LE, et al. A community-based study of explanatory factors for the excess risk for early renal function decline in blacks vs. whites with diabetes: the Atherosclerosis Risk in Communities study. Arch Intern Med 1999;159(5):1777–83.

[12] Klag MJ, Stamler J, Brancat FL, et al. End-stage renal disease in African-American and white men: 16-year MRFIT findings. JAMA 1997;277(16):1293–8.

[13] Coresh J, Wei GK, McQuillian G, et al. Prevalence of high blood pressure and elevated serum creatinine level in the United States: findings from the Third National Health and Nutrition Examination Survey (1988–1994). Arch Intern Med 2001;161:1207–16.

[14] Grim CE, Henry JP, Myers H. High blood pressure in blacks: salt, slavery, survival, stress, and racism. In: Laragh JH, Brenner BM, editors. Hypertension: pathophysiology, diagnosis, and management. New York: Raven Press; 1995. p. 171–207.

[15] US Renal Data System. USRDS 2001 annual data report. Bethesda (MD): National Institutes of Health, National Institute of Diabetes and Digestive and Kidney Diseases; 2001.

[16] Burt VI, Whelton P, Roccalla EJ, et al. Prevalence of hypertension in the US adult population: results from the Third National Health and Nutrition Examination survey 1988–1991. Hypertension 1995;25:305–13.

[17] United Network for Organ Sharing. UNOS 1999 annual report of the US Scientific Registry of Transplant Recipients and the Organ Procurement and Transplantation Network. Transplant data: 1994–1998. Richmond (VA): United Network for Organ Sharing; 1999.

[18] Fogo A, Breyer JA, Smith MC, et al, and the AASK Pilot Study Investigators. Accuracy of the diagnosis of hypertensive nephrosclerosis in African Americans: a report from the African-American Study of Kidney Diseases (AASK) Trial. Kidney Int 1997;51:244–52.

[19] Fogo A, Breyer JA, Smith MC, et al, and AASK Pilot Study Investigators Renal histopathology in US African Americans with presumed hypertensive nephrosclerosis. Nephrology 1998;4:S54–8.

[20] Bergman S, Key BO, Kirk KA, et al. Kidney disease in the first-degree relatives of African Americans with hypertensive end-stage renal disease. Am J Kidney Dis 1996;27:341–6.

[21] Warnock DG. Low renin hypertension in the next millennium. Semin Nephrol 2000;20: 40–6.

[22] Summerson JH, Bell RA, Konen JC. Racial differences in the prevalence of micro-albuminuria in hypertension. Am J Kidney Dis 1995;26:577–9.

[23] Geiger HJ. Race and health care—an American dilemma. New Engl J Med 1996;335:815–6.

[24] Gornick ME, Eggers PW, Reilly TW, et al. Effects of race and income on mortality and use of services among Medicare beneficiaries. New Engl J Med 1996;335:791–9.

[25] Schlessinger SD, Tankersley MR, Curtis JJ. Clinical documentation of end-stage renal disease due to hypertension. Am J Kidney Dis 1994;23:655–60.

[26] Friedman EA, Delano BG, Butt KMH. Pragmatic realities in uremia therapy. N Engl J Med 1978;298:368–71.

[27] Kasiske BL, Cohen D, Lucey MR, et al. Payment for immunosuppression after organ transplantation. JAMA 2000;283:2445–50.

[28] Laupacis A, Keown P, Pus N, et al. A study of the quality of life and cost-utility of renal transplantation. Kidney Int 1996;50:235–42.

[29] Ojo AO, Port FK, Wolfe RA, et al. Comparative mortality risks of chronic dialysis and cadaveric transplantation in black end-stage renal disease patients. Am J Kidney Dis 1994; 24:59–64.

[30] United Network for Organ Sharing. 1998 Annual report—Scientific Registry. Richmond (VA): United Network for Organ Sharing; 1999.

[31] US Renal Data System. USRDS 2002 annual data report. Bethesda (MD): National Institutes of Health, National Institute of Diabetes and Digestive and Kidney Diseases; 2002.

[32] Thamer M, Hwang W, Fink NE, et al. US nephrologists' attitudes towards renal transplantation: results from a national survey. Transplantation 2001;71(2):281–8.

[33] Soucie JM, Neylan JF, McClellan W. Race and sex differences in the identification of candidates for renal transplantation. Am J Kidney Dis 1992;19:414–9.

[34] Ayanian JZ, Clearly PD, Keogh JH, et al. Physician's beliefs about racial differences in referral for renal transplantation. Am J Kidney Dis 2004;43(2):350–7.

[35] Ayanian JZ, Cleary PD, Weissman JS, et al. The effect of patients' preferences on racial differences in access to renal transplantation. New Engl J Med 1999;341:1661–9.

[36] Epstein AM, Ayanian JZ, Keogh JH, et al. Racial disparities in access to renal transplantation. N Engl J Med 2000;343(21):1537–44.

[37] Kallich JD, Adams JL, Barton PL, et al. Access to cadaveric kidney transplantation. Santa Monica (CA): Rand/UCLA/Harvard Center for Health Care Financing Policy Research; 1993.

[38] Garg PP, Diener-West M, Powe NR. Reducing racial disparities in transplant activation: whom should we target? Am J Kidney Dis 2001;37(5):921–31.

[39] Tankersley MR, Gaston RS, Curtis JJ, et al. The living donor process in kidney transplantation: influence of race and co-morbidity. Transplant Proc 1997;29:3722–3.

[40] Kasiske BL, London W, Ellison M. Race and socioeconomic factors influencing early placement on the kidney transplant waiting list. J Am Soc Nephrol 1998;9:2142–7.

[41] Meier-Kriesche HU, Port FK, Ojo AO, et al. Effect of waiting time on renal transplant outcome. Kidney Int 2000;58:1311–7.

[42] Kerman RH, Kimball PM, Van Buren CT, et al. Influence of race on crossmatch outcome and recipient eligibility for transplantation. Transplantation 1992;53:64–7.

[43] Norman DJ, Ellison MD, Breen TJ, et al. Cadaveric kidney allocation in the United States: a critical analysis of the point system. Transplant Proc 1995;27:800.

[44] Lazda VA, Blaesing ME. Is allocation of kidneys on basis of HLA match equitable in multiracial populations? Transplant Proc 1989;21:1415–6.

[45] Lazda VA. The impact of HLA frequency differences in races on the access to optimally HLA-matched cadaver renal transplants. Transplantation 1992;53:352–7.

[46] Barger B, Shroyer TW, Hudson SL, et al. The impact of the UNOS mandatory sharing policy on recipients of the black and white races: experience at a single renal transplant center. Transplantation 1992;53:770–4.

[47] Takemoto SK, Terasaki PI, et al. Twelve years' experience with national sharing of HLA matched cadaveric kidneys for transplantation. New Engl J Med 2000;343(15): 1078–84.

[48] Hata Y, Ozawa M, Takemoto SK, et al. HLA matching. In: Cecka JM, Terasaki PI, editors. Clinical transplants 1996. Los Angeles (CA): UCLA Tissue Typing Laboratory; 1997. p. 381–96.

[49] Scantlebury V, Gjertson D, Eliasziw M, et al. Effect of HLA mismatch in African Americans. Transplantation 1998;65:586–8.

[50] Takemoto S, Terasaki PI, Gjertson DW, et al. Equitable allocation of HLA-compatible kidneys for local pools and for minorities. New Engl J Med 1994;331:760–4.

[51] Takemoto S, Terasaki PI, Cecka JM, et al. For the UNOS Renal Transplant Registry. Survival of nationally shared, HLA-matched kidney transplants from cadaveric donors. New Engl J Med 1992;327:834–9.

[52] Cecka JM. The UNOS Scientific Renal Transplant Registry. In: Cecka JM, Terasaki PI, editors. Clinical transplants 1998. Los Angeles (CA): UCLA Tissue Typing Laboratory; 1999. p. 1–16.

[53] Gjertson DW. Short- and long-term effects of HLA matching. In: Terasaki PI, editor. Clinical transplants 1989. Los Angeles (CA): UCLA Tissue Typing Laboratory; 1989. p. 353–60.

[54] Gjertson DW. Two-factor reference tables for renal transplantation. In: Cecka JM, Terasaki PI, editors. Clinical transplants 1995. Los Angeles (CA): UCLA Tissue Typing Laboratory; 1996. p. 433–85.

[55] Held PJ, Kahan BD, Hunsicker LG, et al. The impact of HLA mismatches on the survival of first cadaveric kidney transplants. New Engl J Med 1994;331:765–70.

[56] Feldman HI, Roth DA, Fazio I, et al. National kidney allograft sharing: a decision analysis. Transplantation 1997;64:80–8.

[57] Gaston RS, Ayres I, Dooley LG, et al. Racial equity in renal transplantation: the disparate impact of HLA-based allocation. JAMA 1993;270:1352–6.

[58] Scaife ER, Mone MC, Shelby J, et al. Characteristics of kidneys offered as paybacks in the zero-antigen mismatch sharing policy. Transplant Proc 1997;29:3441–3.

[59] United Network for Organ Sharing. Point change results from UNOS study. Richmond (VA): United Network for Organ Sharing; Update 1994; Dec:18.

[60] Delmonico FL, Milford EL, Goguen J, et al. A novel United Network for Organ Sharing region kidney allocation plan improves transplant access for minority candidates. Transplantation 1999;68:1875–9.

[61] Chertow GM, Brenner BM, Mackenzie HS, et al. Non-immunologic predictors of chronic renal allograft failure: data from the United Network for Organ Sharing. Kidney Int 1995; 52(Suppl 52):S48–51.

[62] Halloran PF, Melk A, Barth C. Rethinking chronic allograft nephropathy: the concept of accelerated senescence. J Am Soc Nephrol 1999;10:167–81.

[63] Ojo AO, Wolfe RA, Held PJ, et al. Delayed graft function: risk factors and implications for renal allograft survival. Transplantation 1997;63:968–74.

[64] Schweitzer EJ, Yoon S, Hart J, et al. Increased living donor volunteer rates with a formal recipient family education program. Am J Kidney Dis 1997;29:739–45.

[65] Ojo A, Port FK. Influence of race and gender on related donor renal transplantation rates. Am J Kidney Dis 1993;22:835–41.

[66] Ratner LE, Ciseck LJ, Moore RG, et al. Laparoscopic live donor nephrectomy. Transplantation 1995;60:1047–9.

[67] Barger BO, Hudson SL, Shroyer TW, et al. Influence of race on renal allograft survival in the pre and post-cyclosporine era. In: Terasaki PI, editor. Clinical transplants 1987. Los Angeles (CA): UCLA Tissue Typing Laboratory; 1987. p. 217–33.

[68] Ojo AO, Port FK, Held PJ, et al. Inferior outcome of two-haplotype matched renal transplants in blacks: role of early rejection. Kidney Int 1995;48:1592–9.

[69] Opelz G, Pfarr E, Engelmann A, et al. Kidney graft survival rates in black cyclosporine-treated patients. Transplant Proc 1989;21:3918–20.

[70] Katznelson S, Gjertson DW, Cecka JM. The effect of race and ethnicity on kidney allograft outcome. In: Cecka JM, Terasaki PI, editors. Clinical transplants 1995. Los Angeles (CA): UCLA Tissue Typing Laboratory; 1996. p. 379–94.

[71] Gaston RS, Hudson SL, Deierhoi MH, et al. Improved survival of primary cadaveric renal allografts in blacks with quadruple immunosuppression. Transplantation 1992;53: 103–9.

[72] Yuge J, Cecka JM. The race effect. In: Terasaki PI, editor. Clinical transplants 1989. Los Angeles (CA): UCLA Tissue Typing Laboratory; 1989. p. 407–15.

[73] Oplez G, Wujciak T, Ritz E. Association of chronic kidney graft failure with recipient blood pressure. Collaborative Transplant Study. Kidney Int 1998;53(1):217–22.

[74] Cosio FG, Dillon JJ, Falkenhain ME, et al. Racial differences in renal allograft survival: the role of systemic hypertension. Kidney Int 1995;47:1136–41.

[75] Martinez-Castelao A, Hueso M, Sanz V, et al. treatment of hypertension after renal transplantation: long-term efficacy of verapamil, enalapril, and doxazosin. Kidney Int 1998;54(Suppl):S130–4.

[76] Curtis JJ. Management of hypertension. Kidney Int 1993;43(Suppl):S45–9.

[77] Messerli FH. Hypertension in special populations. Med Clin N Am 1997;81:1335–45.

[78] Weinberger MH. Hypertension in African Americans: the role of sodium chloride and extracellular fluid volume. Semin Nephrol 1996;16:110–6.

[79] Falkner B. The role of cardiovascular reactivity as a mediator of hypertension in African Americans. Semin Nephrol 1996;16:117–25.

[80] Grubbs AL, Ergul A. A review of endothelin and hypertension in African Americans individuals. Ethn Dis 2001;11:741–8.

[81] The Sixth Report of the Joint National Committee on Prevention. Detection, Evaluation, and Treatment of High Blood Pressure. Bethesda (MD)· National Institutes of Health, National Heart, Lung, and Blood Institute; 1997.

[82] Wright JT Jr, Kusek JW, Toto RD, et al. Design and baseline characteristics of participants in the African American Study of Kidney Disease and Hypertension (AASK) Pilot Study. Control Clin Trials 1996;17:3S–16S.

[83] Agodoa LY, Appel L, Bakris GL, et al, for the African-American Study of Kidney Disease and Hypertension (AASK) Study Group. Effect of ramipril vs. amlodipine on renal outcomes in hypertensive nephrosclerosis. A randomized controlled trial. JAMA 2001;285: 2719–28.

[84] Wright JT Jr, Bakris G, Greene T, et al, for the African-American Study of Kidney Disease and Hypertension Study Group. Effect of blood pressure lowering and anti-hypertensive

drug class on progression of hypertensive kidney disease: results of the AASK Trial. JAMA 2001;282:2421–31.

[85] Winston JS, Burns GC, Klotman PE. The human immunodeficiency virus (HIV) epidemic and HIV-associated nephropathy. Semin Nephrol 1998;18(4):373–7.

[86] Woodward RS, Schnitzler MA, Lowell JA, et al. Medicare's extended immunosuppression coverage improved graft survival [abstract]. J Am Soc Nephrol 1999;10:751A.

[87] Anonymous. Latino Americans: the face of the future. Newsweek. July 12, 1999:50–1.

[88] Schweizer RT, Rovelli M, Palmeri D, et al. Noncompliance in organ transplant recipients. Transplantation 1990;49:374–7.

[89] Curtis JJ. Kidney transplantation: racial or socioeconomic disparities? Am J Kidney Dis 1999;34:756–8.

[90] Isaacs RB, Nock S, Spencer C, et al. Racial disparities in renal transplant outcomes. Am J Kidney Dis 1999;34:706–12.

[91] Didlake RH, Dreyfus K, Kerman RH, et al. Patient non-compliance: a major cause of late graft failure in cyclosporine-treated renal transplants. Transplant Proc 1988;20:63.

[92] Gaston RS, Hudson SL, Ward M, et al. Late renal allograft loss: non-compliance masquerading as chronic rejection. Transplant Proc 1999;31(Suppl 4A):21S.

[93] Kalil RSN, Heiem-Duthoy KL, Kasiski BL. Patients with low income have reduced renal allograft survival. Am J Kidney Dis 1992;20(1):63–9.

[94] Butkus DE, Dottes AL, Meydrech E, et al. Effect of poverty and other socioeconomic variables on renal allograft survival. Transplantation 2002;72(2):261–6.

[95] Isaacs RB, Conners A, Nock S, et al. Noncompliance in living-related donor renal transplantation: the United Network of Organ Sharing Experience. Transplantation Proc 1999;31(Suppl 4A):19S–20S.

[96] Sanders CE, Curtis JJ, Julian BA, et al. Tapering or discontinuing cyclosporine for financial reasons—a single center experience. Am J Kidney Dis 1993;21:9–15.

[97] Sanders CE, Julian BA, Gaston RS, et al. Benefits of continued cyclosporine through an indigent drug program. Am J Kidney Dis 1996;28:572–7.

[98] Gaston RS. Evolution of Medicare policy involving transplantation and immunosuppressive medications: past developments and future directions. In: Field MJ, Lawrence RL, Zwanziger L, editors. Extending Medicare coverage for preventive and other services. Washington, DC: National Academy Press; 2000. p. 310–28.

[99] Oliver JD, Yuan CM, Welch PG, et al. Renal allograft survival is independent of race in the US Military Health Care System [abstract]. J Am Soc Nephrol 1999;10:741A.

[100] Emovon OE, King JAC, Holt CO, et al. Effect of cyclosporine pharmacokinetics on renal allograft outcome in African Americans. Clin Transplant 2003;17:206–11.

[101] International Neoral Renal Transplantation Study Group. Randomized, international study of cyclosporine microemulsion absorption profiling in renal transplantation with basiliximab immunoprophylaxis. Am J Transplant 2002;2:157–66.

[102] Neylan JF. Racial differences in renal transplantation after immunosuppression with tacrolimus versus cyclosporine. Transplantation 1998;65(4):515–23.

[103] Andrews PA, Sen M, Chang RW. Racial variations in dosage requirements of tacrolimus [letter]. Lancet 1996;348:1446.

[104] Heifets M, Cooney G, Shaw L, et al., Ethnic differences in tacrolimus pharmacokinetics in renal transplant candidates. 1996 Annual Meeting of the American Society of Transplant Physicians. Abstracts-On-Disk: K-KT-099.

[105] Macphee IAM, Fredericks S, Tai T, et al. Tacrolimus pharmacogenetics: polymorphisms associated with expression of cytochrome P4503A5 and p-glycoprotein correlate with dose requirement. Transplantation 2002;74(11):1486–9.

[106] Thervet E, Anglicheau D, King B, et al. Impact of cytochrome P450 genetic polymorphism on tacrolimus doses and concentration-to-dose ratio in renal transplant recipients. Transplantation 2003;76(8):1233–5.

[107] Tsuchiya N, Satoh S, Tada H, et al. Influence of CYP3A5 and MDR1(ABCB1) polymorphisms on the pharmacokinetics of tacrolimus in renal transplant recipients. Transplantation 2004;78(8):1182–7.

[108] Leffell MS, Steinberg AG, Bias WB, et al. The distribution of HLA antigens and phenotypes among donors and patients in the UNOS registry. Transplantation 1994;58:1119–30.

[109] Zhou YC, Cecka JM, Terasaki PI. Effect of race on kidney transplants. In: Terasaki PI, editor. Clinical transplants 1990. Los Angeles (CA): UCLA Tissue Typing Laboratory; 1991. p. 447–59.

[110] Oplez G, Mytilineos J, Scherer S, et al. Influence of HLA matching and DNA typing on kidney and heart transplant survival in black recipients. Transplant Proc 1997;29:3333–5.

[111] Port FK, Ashby VB, Leichtman AB, et al. Eliminating points for HLA-B similarity increased allocation to minority, pediatric, sensitized, and zero MM candidates [abstract]. American Journal of Transplantation 2004;4(8):414–41.

[112] Rebellato LM, Arnold AN, Bozik KM, et al. HLA matching and the united network for organ sharing allocation system: impact of HLA matching on African-American recipients of cadaveric kidney transplants. Transplantation 2002;74(11):1634–6.

[113] Mottram PL, Han WR, Purcell LJ, et al. Increased expression of IL-4 and IL-10 and decreased expression of IL-2 and interferon-γ in long-surviving mouse heart allografts after brief CD-4 monoclonal antibody therapy. Transplantation 1995;59:559–65.

[114] Minguela A, Torio A, Marin L, et al. Implication of Th1, Th2, and Th3 cytokines in liver graft acceptance. Transplant Proc 1993;31:519–20.

[115] Wilson AG, Symons JA, McDowell TL, et al. Effects of a polymorphism in the human tumor necrosis factor a (TNF-α) promoter in transcriptional activation. Proc Natl Acad Sci U S A 1997;94:3195–9.

[116] Fuggle SV, Koo DD. Cell adhesion molecules in clinical renal transplantation. Transplantation 1998;65:763–9.

[117] Halloran PF, Broski AP, Batiuk TD, et al. the molecular immunology of acute rejection: an overview. Transplant Immunol 1993;1:3–27.

[118] Suthanthiran M. Acute rejection of renal allografts; mechanistic insights and therapeutic options. Kidney Int 1997;51:1289–304.

[119] Bathgate AJ, Pravica V, Perry C, et al. The effect of polymorphism in tumor necrosis factor-α, interleukine-10, and transforming growth factor-$\beta1$ genes in acute hepatic allograft rejection. Transplantation 2000;69:1514–7.

[120] Sankaran D, Asderakis A, Asharf S, et al. Cytokine gene polymorphisms predict acute graft rejection following renal transplantation. Kidney Int 1999;56:281–8.

[121] Hutchinson IV, Pravica V, Sinnott P. Genetic regulation of cytokine synthesis; consequences for acute and chronic organ allograft rejection. Graft 2000;56:281.

[122] Suthanthiran M. The importance of genetic polymorphisms in renal transplantation. Curr Opin Urol 2000;10(2):71–5.

[123] Asderakis A, Sanaran D, Dyer P, et al. Association of polymorphisms in the human interferon-γ and interleukin-10 gene with acute and chronic kidney transplant outcome. The cytokine effect on transplantation. Transplantation 2001;71:674–8.

[124] Hutchinson IV, Turner D, Sankaran D, et al. Cytokine genotypes in allograft rejection: guidelines for immunosuppression. Transplant Proc 1998;30:3991–2.

[125] Wilson AG, di Giovine FS, Blakemore AI, et al. Single base polymorphism in the human tumor necrosis factor-α (TNF-α) gene detectable by Ncol restriction of PCR product. Hum Mol Genet 1992;1(5):353.

[126] John S, Turner D, Donn R, et al. Two novel bi-allelic polymorphisms in the IL-2 gene. Eur J Immunogenet 1998;25:419–20.

[127] McDaniel DO, Barber WH, Nguyan C, et al. Combined analysis of cytokine genotype polymorphism and the level of expression with allograft function in African-American renal transplant patients. Transplant Immunol 2002;11:107–19.

[128] Hutchings A, Purcell WM, Benfield MR. Increased co-stimulatory responses in African American kidney allograft recipients. Transplantation 2001;71(5):692–5.

[129] Azuma H, Chandraker A, Nedeau K, et al. Blockade of T-cell co-stimulation prevents development of experimental chronic renal allograft rejection. Proc Natl Acad Sci U S A 1996;93(22):12439–44.

[130] Pearson TC, Alexander DZ, Corbascio M, et al. Analysis of the B7 co-stimulatory pathway in allograft rejection. Transplantation 1997;63(10):1463.

[131] Kerman RH, Kimball PM, Van Buren CT, et al. Possible contribution of pretransplant immune responder status to renal allograft survival differences of black versus white recipients. Transplantation 1991;51:338–42.

[132] Neylan JF. Immunosuppressive therapy in high-risk transplant patients: dose-dependent efficacy of mycophenolate mofetil in African-American renal allograft recipients. Transplantation 1997;64:1277–82.

[133] Meier-Kriesche HU, Ojo AO, Leichtman AB, et al. Effect of mycophenolate mofetil on long-term outcomes in African American renal transplant recipients. J Am Soc Nephrol 2000;11:2366–70.

[134] Hricik DE, Anton HA, Knauss TC, et al. Outcomes of African American kidney transplant recipients with sirolimus, tacrolimus, and corticosteroids. Transplantation 2002;74(2): 189–93.

[135] Klassen AC, Hall AG, Saksvig B, et al. Relationship between patient's perceptions of disadvantage and discrimination and listing for kidney transplantation. Am J Public Health 2002;92(5):811–7.

[136] Cooper-Patrick L, Gallo JJ, Gonzales JJ, et al. Race, gender, and partnership in the patient-physician relationship. JAMA 1999;282:583–9.

[137] Sculman KA, Berlin JA, Harless W, et al. The effect of race and sex on physician's recommendations for cardiac catheterization. New Engl J Med 1999;340:618–26.

[138] Zachary AA, Braun WE, Hayes JM, et al. Effect of HLA matching on organ distribution among whites and African Americans. Transplantation 1994;57:1115–9.

[139] Harper AM, Rosendale JD, McBride MA, et al. The UNOS OPTN waiting list and donor registry. In: Cecka JM, Terasaki PI, editors. Clinical transplants 1998. Los Angeles (CA): UCLA Tissue Typing Laboratory; 1999. p. 73–90.

[140] Callender C, Burston B, Yeager C, et al. A national minority transplant program for increasing donation rates. Transplant Proc 1997;29:1482–3.

[141] Hricik DE, Whalen CC, Lautman J, et al. Withdrawal of steroids after renal transplantation-clinical predictors of outcome. Transplantation 1992;53:41–5.

[142] Matas A, Ewell M. Prednisone withdrawal in kidney transplant recipients on CsA/MMF- a prospective, randomized study [abstract]. Transplantation 1999;67:S269.

[143] Koyama H, Cecka JM, Terasaki PI. Kidney transplants in black recipients: HLA matching and other factors affecting long-term graft survival. Transplantation 1994;57:1064–8.

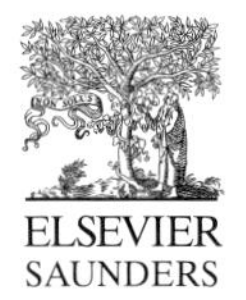

THE MEDICAL
CLINICS
OF NORTH AMERICA

Med Clin N Am 89 (2005) 1033–1043

Is There Disparity in the Care of Minority Patients with Upper Aerodigestive Tract Malignancy?

Cheryl L. Walker, MD[a], Pablo Mojica-Manosa, MD[b], Wesley L. Hicks, Jr, MD[b], Wade Douglas, MD[b], Billy R. Ballard, MD[c], Nestor R. Rigual, MD[b], Sharon Spencer, MD[d],*

[a]The Kerr L. White Institute for Health Services Research, 6555 Sugarloaf Parkway, Suite 307-121, Duluth, GA 30097, USA
[b]Department of Head and Neck Surgery, Roswell Park Cancer Institute, Elm and Carlton Streets, Buffalo, NY 14263, USA
[c]Department of Pathology, Anatomy, and Cell Biology, Meharry Medical College, 1005 D.B. Todd Boulevard, Nashville, TN 37208, USA
[d]Head and Neck Oncology, Department of Radiation, University of Alabama at Birmingham School of Medicine, 619 19th Street South, Birmingham, AL 35233-1924, USA

Cancer is second only to heart disease as a cause of death. It is characterized by unregulated growth and spread of abnormal cells [1]. According to the Surveillance, Epidemiology and End Results (SEER) data, approximately 1.4 million people in the United States were diagnosed with a malignancy in 2004. Of those, 563,700 persons are expected to die [2]. The National Cancer database (from 1985–1995) reported that cancer of the head and neck represented 6.6% of all malignancies registered [3].

The upper aerodigestive tract consists of the nasal cavity, paranasal sinuses, nasopharynx, middle ear, oral cavity, lips, pharynx, larynx, cervical esophagus, and salivary and thyroid glands. In the United States approximately 38,430 new head and neck cancers were reported in 2004 and 11,060 (29%) will succumb to their disease [2]. A total of 28,260 patients with cancer of the oral cavity and pharynx are expected to succumb to the disease. A total of 10,270 patients with cancer of the larynx are expected to die [2]. The 5-year survival rate for the most common malignancy of the

---

* Corresponding author.
E-mail address: sspencer@uabmc.edu (S. Spencer).

aerodigestive tract (squamous cell carcinoma) has varied from 50% to 60% over the last 30 years.

The incidence of head and neck squamous cell carcinoma (HNSCC) in African-American men is twice that of whites, whereas the rate for African-American women parallels that of white women. In 1998, the first documented decline in cancer death rate was noted since United States reporting began [4]. Overall incidence rates declined 0.5% per year from 1995 to 2001 and stabilized for all races. The mortality rate also decreased over 1993 to 2001. All races and ethnic groups saw a decrease by 1.1% per year from 1993 to 2001 [4]. Despite these encouraging reports, African Americans have the highest incidence and death rate from all HNSCC cancer sites combined [4].

Primary tumor location and stage at the time of presentation are important determinates of survival. Upper aerodigestive tract carcinomas often have vague presenting symptoms and can present initially at an advanced stage. Patients with HNSCC presenting in the oral cavity and hypopharynx typically have a worse outcome versus patients who present with cancers in the larynx. The SEER has shown a 5-year relative survival rate of 68% for the larynx and 57% for the oral cavity and pharynx from 1995 to 2000 for men [4]. Interestingly women, unlike their male counterparts, had a 60% 5-year survival rate for larynx and 61.5% rate for oral cavity and the pharynx.

African-American men typically have a higher incidence in those head and neck subsites that are known to have less favorable outcomes (Tables 1–3). Single institution data seem to confirm the trends seen nationally (Table 4) [5]. African Americans also present with localized disease less often than other ethnic populations (Tables 5–9). According to the American Cancer Society statistics for 2003, 19% of oral cavity and pharyngeal cases in African Americans are localized at the time of diagnosis versus 34% for all groups and 37% for whites. These differences are also reflected in the 5-year survival rates for patients. The relative 5-year survival rate from 1992 to 1998 was 68% for African Americans versus 82% for all other ethnic populations [2]. There are no data suggesting different biologic behavior in squamous cell cancer in African-American patients; however, there is evidence suggesting that the different and often poorer clinical outcomes

Table 1

Surveillance, Epidemiology, and End Results incidence rates 1992–2001

Sex	All	African Americans	Whites
Males			
Oral cavity	16.7	21.4	16.5
Larynx	7.3	12.9	7.2
Females			
Oral cavity	6.7	6.5	6.7
Larynx	—	—	—

Data from Jemal A, Clegg LX, Ward E, et al. Annual report to the nation on the status of cancer, 1975–2001, with a special feature regarding survival. Cancer 2004;101(1):3–27.

Table 2
National Program of Cancer Registries and Surveillance, Epidemiology, and End Results registries: age adjusted invasive cancer incidence rates 2000

Location	All	African Americans	Whites
Larynx	1.6	2.2	1.6
Oral cavity/pharynx	6.0	5.1	6.0
Thyroid	10.7	6.7	11.0
Lip	0.3	—	0.3
Tongue	1.5	1.0	1.6
Salivary gland	0.9	0.6	0.9
Floor of mouth	0.4	0.4	0.4
Gums/other mouth	1.3	1.2	1.3
Nasopharynx	0.3	0.4	0.3
Tonsil	0.5	0.5	0.5
Oropharynx	0.2	0.3	0.3
Hypopharynx	0.3	0.4	0.3
Other oral cavity/pharynx	0.2	0.3	0.2
Nose, nasal cavity/middle ear	0.5	0.4	0.5

Rate per 100,000 person and age-adjusted females.

Data from Surveillance, Epidemiology, and End Results: 2000. Available at: http://aapsneed.cdc.gov/uscs/index.

seen in minority patients are caused by multiple medical, social, and access issues resulting in disparate care for minority patients.

Risk factors in minority groups

Squamous cell carcinoma is the most common type of head and neck cancer. Among the risk factors associated with this type of cancer, tobacco

Table 3
National Program of Cancer Registries and Surveillance, Epidemiology, and End Results registries: age-adjusted invasive cancer incidence rate 2000

Location	All	African Americans	Whites
Larynx	7.0	7.6	7.2
Oral cavity/pharynx	14.5	12.7	14.9
Thyroid	3.6	1.6	3.9
Lip	1.3	0.1	1.5
Tongue	3.5	2.6	3.7
Salivary gland	1.44	2.6	3.7
Floor of mouth	1.1	1.4	1.1
Gums/other mouth	1.8	1.8	1.8
Nasopharynx	0.8	0.9	0.6
Tonsil	2.2	1.9	2.3
Oropharynx	0.6	0.8	0.6
Hypopharynx	1.3	1.9	1.3
Other oral cavity/pharynx	0.5	0.7	0.5
Nose, nasal cavity/middle ear	0.8	0.6	0.8

Rate per 100,000 person and age-adjusted males.

Data from Surveillance, Epidemiology, and End Results: 2000. Available at: http://aapsneed.cdc.gov/uscs/index.

Table 4
Head and neck incidence

Location	All (%)	African Americans (%)	Whites (%)
Oral cavity	554 (61)	49 (52)	505 (62)
Pharynx	355 (39)	45 (48)	310 (38)

MD Anderson Series, N = 909.
Data from Moore RJ, Doherty DA, Do K-A, et al. Racial disparity in survival of patients with squamous cell carcinoma of the oral cavity and pharynx. Ethn Health 2001;6:165–77.

use is the most important. Alcohol abuse is a risk factor that demonstrates a synergistic effect with tobacco use.

Cigarette smoking has been shown to be associated with an increased risk of HNSCC with a fourfold risk in some studies [6–10]. The risk increases with the length of time the individual smoked [6,11]. The daily consumption and lifetime consumption have also been shown to play a role in cancer risk [12]. There is evidence that a history of cigarette smoking versus nonsmokers is associated with a difference in survival for patients with head and neck cancer with a threefold increased risk of death [13].

Differences in cigarette smoking and alcohol consumption have been cited as contributing factors to increased cancer incidence in minorities. Twenty-four and a half percent of all adults are current smokers, which are defined as smoking 100 cigarettes and current. Native Americans have the highest cigarette-smoking rate (37.9%), followed by African Americans (29%), whites (27%), and Hispanics (19%, with Puerto Ricans most likely at 25.8%). Oral cavity and pharynx cancer incidence is higher in African Americans than whites (17.7% compared with 14.8%). In contrast, Hispanics and Asian and Pacific Islanders have a lower incidence of cancers of the oral cavity and pharynx (9.7% and 9%, respectively).

The increased smoking observed among African Americans might in part be a result of increased advertising targeting their communities. Tobacco billboards are in higher densities in racial and ethnic communities. In one study conducted in California, Los Angeles had the highest density of tobacco billboards in the African-American communities and the lowest in the white communities [14]. Publications targeting the African-American

Table 5
Oral cavity and pharynx: age-adjusted Surveillance, Epidemiology, and End Results incidence and US death rates 1997–2001

Race	Total	Male	Female
African-American	4.3	7.5	2.0
White	2.6	3.9	1.6
All	2.8	4.3	1.6

Rates per 100,000 persons.
Data from Surveillance, Epidemiology, and End Results. National Cancer Institute SEER Cancer Statistics review 1975–2001. Available at: http://seer.cancer.gov/csr_1975-2001.

Table 6
Larynx: age-adjusted Surveillance, Epidemiology, and End Results incidence and US death rates 1997–2001

Race	Total	Male	Female
African-American	2.7	5.4	0.9
White	1.3	2.3	0.5
All	1.4	2.6	0.5

Rates per 100,000 persons.

Data from Surveillance, Epidemiology, and End Results. National Cancer Institute SEER Cancer Statistics review 1975–2001. Available at: http://seer.cancer.gov/csr_1975-2001.

public are more likely to have cigarette advertisements than publications targeting the general public. One study found that three major African-American publications, *Ebony*, *Jet*, and *Essence*, had 12% more cigarette advertisements than widespread publications like *Newsweek*, *Time*, *People*, and *Mademoiselle* [15].

Cigarette smoking also varies by geographic location and socioeconomic class. High prevalence of current smoking states includes North Carolina, Kentucky, West Virginia, North Carolina, and Tennessee. Low prevalence areas include Utah, Puerto Rico, California, and Hawaii [16]. Other factors associated with increased rate of cigarette smoking include low socioeconomic status and high school education.

Smoking habits among ethnic groups differ. More African Americans smoke mentholated cigarettes, which contain higher carbon monoxide concentration and may have greater nicotine absorption [17]. The Surgeon General's report from 1998 showed that members of racial ethnic groups tend to participate less in cessation programs than whites [18].

The prevalence of marijuana in the United States has been studied [19]. Two large studies, one conducted during 1991 to 1992 and the other from 2001 to 2002, showed that there was an increased use of marijuana in specific ethnic groups. The largest increase was noted in young African-American men and women and among young Hispanic men [19]. The use of marijuana has been associated with squamous cell cancer of the head and neck. One study from the University of California at Los Angeles reported

Table 7
Stage at diagnosis, 1992–1998: oral cavity and pharynx

Staging	White (%)	African-American (%)	All (%)
Localized	37	19	34
Regional	44	55	46
Distant	8	9	9

Data from Jemal A, Murray T, Samuel A, et al. Cancer facts and figures 2004. National Cancer Institute Surveillance, Epidemiology and End Results Program. National Center for Health Statistics, Centers for Disease Control and Prevention; 2003. CA Cancer J Clin 2003;53:5–26.

Table 8
Relative 5-year survival 1992–1998: oral cavity and pharynx

Staging	White (%)	African-American (%)	All (%)
Localized	82	68	82
Regional	49	29	47
Distant	24	19	23
All Stages	59	35	56

Data from Jemal A, Murray T, Samuel A, et al. Cancer facts and figures 2004. National Cancer Institute Surveillance, Epidemiology and End Results Program. National Center for Health Statistics, Centers for Disease Control and Prevention; 2003. CA Cancer J Clin 2003;53:5–26.

a 2.6% increase risk of squamous cell cancer of the head and neck in persons who used marijuana versus those who never smoked, after controlling for age, gender, race, education, alcohol consumption, cigarette smoking, and passive smoking [20].

Alcohol is associated with increased risk of developing squamous cell cancer of the head and neck when adjusted for cigarette smoking [21–25]. This association has been studied primarily in whites [26], making comparisons with minority groups more difficult. Historically, African Americans have been reported as heavy consumers of alcohol that is attributed to "social disorganization." Recent studies, however, contrast stereotypes regarding African-American alcohol consumption. African-American women are more likely to abstain from alcohol than white women (55% versus 39%). In the 1995 National Alcohol Survey, black men and white men reported similar alcohol consumption between ages 20 and 49. Between ages 50 and 59, white men are more likely to report a higher consumption. African Americans were also more likely to report alcohol consumption, whereas Native Americans and Pacific Islanders are the most likely to report binge drinking and heavy alcohol use. In 2003, African Americans were less likely to report alcohol use, binge drinking, and heavy alcohol use than whites (54.4%, 37.9%, 23.6%, 19%, 7.7%, and 4.5%, respectively). American Indians, Pacific Islanders, Hispanics, and Asian had similar rates of alcohol use (42%, 43.3%, 41%, and 39.8, respectively). Asians reported a lower rate of binge drinking and heavy alcohol use, however, than Native Americans, Hispanics, and Pacific Islanders.

Table 9
All head and neck sites

Staging	African-American (%)	Hispanic (%)	White (%)	All (%)
Localized	26.4	33.3	39.9	37.5
Regional	51.0	51.9	48.5	49.1
Distant	22.5	14.8	11.5	13.3

Data from Shavers VL, Harlan LC, Winn D, et al. Racial/ethnic patterns of care for cancer of the oral cavity, pharynx, larynx, sinuses and salivary gland. Cancer Metastasis Rev 2003;22:25–38.

Diagnosis

Differences in health care–seeking behaviors, such as use of a primary care physician, use of a dentist, and adherence to recommendations for cancer screening, may contribute to a delay in diagnosis. African Americans, Hispanics, and Asians are less likely to report having a primary care physician than whites. In addition, they may be less likely to present for routine nonacute evaluation. A disproportionate number of African Americans and Hispanics report using the emergency room as their primary source of care. Emergency room physicians do not provide preventive services (Fig. 1).

Dentists most often perform oral examinations and yet, few Americans report having oral cancer examinations. In one survey, only 15% of adults reported having had an oral cancer examination. Adults who were above the poverty level, white, non-Hispanic, 40 to 46 years of age, and who had more than a high school education and a higher level of knowledge about risk factors for oral cancer were more likely to have had an oral cancer examination [27]. African Americans are less likely to have regular dental appointments. Other patient characteristics associated with no recent dental care in African Americans include older age, worse health, not working, no regular medical provider, and no recent mammography [28]. Similarly, Hispanics are 1.7 times less likely than non-Hispanics to report having had an oral cancer examination in the past 12 months [29].

There is also evidence that some dentists are not conducting cancer-screening examinations. One study of Maryland dentist groups was conducted to obtain more in-depth information about why dentists do not provide a comprehensive oral cancer examination for most of their patients. Inaccurate knowledge about oral cancer, inconsistency in oral cancer examinations, lack of confidence in when and how to palpate for

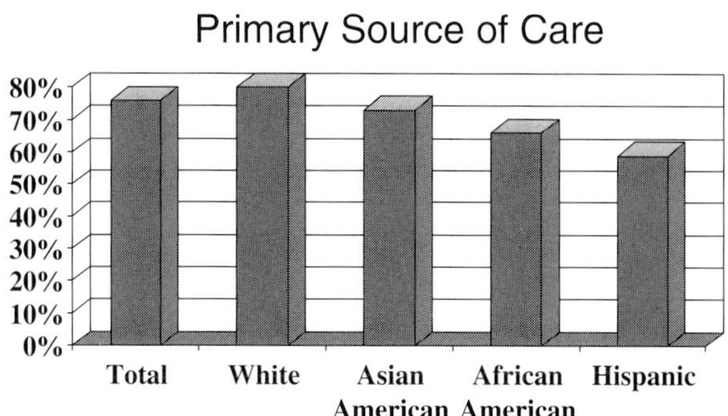

Fig. 1. Percent of adults reporting doctor's office as regular source of care. (*Data from* Diverse communities, common concerns: assessing health care quality for minority Americans. The Commonwealth Fund 2001 Health Quality Survey. Available at: http://www.cmwf.org/surveys/surveys.)

abnormalities, and lack of time routinely to provide oral cancer examinations were reported to be significant factors [30].

Minority patients may not trust the physician or health care system as much as whites, which may negatively influence adherence to recommended screenings, diagnostic evaluations, and even treatments. At the same time, health care providers may interact with minority patients differently, which may be influenced by stereotypes. Health care providers are more likely to recommend more aggressive therapies in white patients than minority patients, even when they have the same insurance coverage and present with the same stage of disease.

Ultimately, the combination of all these factors interplay influencing the diagnosis of HNSCC. Lack of access to health care, low socioeconomic status, and lower education in the minority groups delay the diagnosis and lead to patients presenting with more advance staging.

Staging, treatments, and survival in minority groups

Treatment for HNSCC typically includes radiation, surgery, or a combination of these two modalities. The role of chemotherapy has gained an important part in the treatment strategy in the last decade, being used more often as an adjuvant therapy in combination with radiation or surgery. Ultimately, tumor location and extent of the disease dictate the treatment chosen for each individual patient.

HNSCC rate patterns in minority groups differ from whites. Even within the minority groups, each racial or ethnic group had different patterns of presentation.

Shavers and coworkers [31] have described the pattern of treatment delivery according to race and ethnicity. Their analysis noted disparity in the delivery of cancer-directed surgery. Overall, 67% of whites and 66.9% of Hispanics received cancer-directed surgery compared with only 50.9% of African Americans. Specifically, African Americans were noted to have less cancer-directed surgery and more radiotherapy for oral cavity and pharynx. African Americans, however, received more cancer-directed surgery and less radiation for the larynx than whites and Hispanics. In their study, nearly 17% of African Americans died of HNSCC within 2 years of diagnosis compared with 11.9% of whites. Shavers and coworkers [31] concluded that differences in treatment strategies according to race might play an important factor in survival disparities between groups. Moore and coworkers [5] reported similar results showing disparities in treatment strategies between racial and ethnic groups. In their study, 19% of the African-American population received cancer-directed surgery compared with 37% of whites. After adjusting for race and treatment received, African Americans had a 1.61% increase risk of dying from their disease than whites. The University of Florida also showed that treatment disparities existed between racial and ethnics groups. In addition, their study reported a higher risk of developing metastatic disease in the African-American group. This increased metastatic rate translates ultimately to decreased survival. The SEER database from 1988 to 1993 of patients with HNSCC has shown not only that African Americans were more likely inappropriately to receive definitive radiation therapy, but also more likely to be offered no therapy when compared with white patients with equivalent site and stage of disease [32].

Others studies, however, have reported no differences in survival between different racial and ethnic groups with same stage and treatment strategies. The Radiation Therapy Oncology Group has reviewed survival in multiple phase II and III trials in patients with HNSCC [33,34]. In their report, a racial and ethnic difference was not a significant predictor for survival. A secondary analysis showed that increased overall survival was found in patients who had a higher degree of education, were married, and had a higher income. The Radiation Therapy Oncology Group trials concluded that when patients are adequately staged and uniformly treated, race is not an independent variable for survival.

Summary

The data presently available indicate that there is unequal (disparate) care in patients with head and neck cancer. The reasons for this are likely multifactorial and require further study [35]. Complicating such work is the need for subgroup analysis. For example, Hispanics are not a homogeneous ethnic group; hence, differences in social perception, cultural mores, and available medical resources can be demonstrated that can directly impact care and outcome. Appropriate epidemiologic studies are needed with more underserved minority patients to analyze these differences further and to address such differences.

References

[1] American Cancer Society. Cancer facts & figures for Hispanics/Latinos and African-Americans 2003–2004. Atlanta (GA): American Cancer Society; 2004. CA Cancer J Clin 2004;54:8–29.

[2] Jemal A, Murray T, Samuel A, et al. Cancer facts and figures 2004. National Cancer Institute Surveillance, Epidemiology and End Results Program. National Center for Health Statistics, Centers for Disease Control and Prevention; 2003. CA Cancer J Clin 2003;53:5–26.

[3] Hoffman HT, Karmell LH, Funk GF, et al. The National Cancer Data Base Report on cancer of the head and neck. Arch Otolaryngol Head Neck Surg 1998;124:951–62.

[4] Jemal A, Clegg L, Ward E, et al. Annual report to the nation on the status of cancer, 1975–2001, with a special feature survival. Cancer 2004;101:3–27.

[5] Moore RJ, Doherty DA, Do K-A, et al. Racial disparity in survival of patients with squamous cell carcinoma of the oral cavity and pharynx. Ethn Health 2001;6:165–77.

[6] Lewin F, Norell SE, Johansson H, et al. Smoking tobacco, oral snuff, and alcohol in the etiology of squamous cell carcinoma of the head and neck. Cancer 1998;82:1367–75.

[7] Blot WJ, McLaughlin JK, Winn DM, et al. Smoking and drinking in relation to oral and pharyngeal cancer. Cancer Res 1988;48:3282–7.

[8] Bundgaard T, Wildt J, Frydenberg M, et al. Case-control study of squamous cell cancer of the oral cavity in Denmark. Cancer Causes Control 1995;6:57–67.

[9] Flanders WD, Rothman KJ. Interaction of tobacco and alcohol in laryngeal cancer. Am J Epidemiol 1982;115:371–9.

[10] Rothman K, Keller A. The effect of joint exposure to alcohol and tobacco on risk of cancer of the mouth and pharynx. J Chronic Dis 1972;25:711–6.

[11] Brugere J, Guenel P, Lecterc A, et al. Differential effects of tobacco and alcohol in cancer of the larynx, pharynx and mouth. Cancer 1986;57:391–5.

[12] Tuyns AJ, Esteve J, Raymond L, et al. Cancer of the larynx/hypopharynx, tobacco and alcohol: IARC international case-control study in Turin and Varese (Italy), Zaragoza and Navarra (Spain), Geneva (Switzerland) and Calvados (France). Int J Cancer 1988;41: 483–91.

[13] Pytynia KB, Grant JR, Efzel CJ, et al. Matched-pair analysis of survival of never smokers and ever smokers with squamous cell carcinoma of the head and neck. J Clin Oncol 2004;22: 3981–8.

[14] Stoddard JL, Johnson CA, Boley-Cruz T, et al. Target tobacco markets: outdoors advertising in Los Angeles minority neighbors. Am J Public Health 1997;87:1232–3.

[15] Cummings KM, Giovino G, Mendicino AJ. Cigarette advertising and black-white differences in brand preference. Public Health Rep 1987;102:698–701.

[16] State-specific prevalence of current cigarette smoking among adults, and policies and attitudes about second hand smoke. United States, 2000. MMWR 2005.

[17] Clark PI, Gautam S, Gerson LW. Effects of menthol cigarettes on biochemical markers of smoke exposure among blacks and white smokers. Chest 1996;110:194–8.

[18] US Department of Health and Human Services. Tobacco use among racial/ethnic groups: African-American, American Indians and Alaska Native, Asian-Americans and Pacific Islanders and Hispanics: report of the Surgeon General. Atlanta (GA): US department of Health and Human Services, Centers for Disease Control and Prevention; 1998.

[19] Compton WM, Grant BF, Colliever JD, et al. Prevalence of marijuana use disorders in the United States 1991–1992 and 2001–2002. JAMA 2004;29:2114–21.

[20] Zhang ZF, Morgenstern H, Spitz MR, et al. Marijuana use and increased risk of squamous cell carcinoma of the head and neck. Cancer Epidemiol Biomarkers Prev 1999; 8:1071–8.

[21] Franceschi S, Biloli E, Negri E, et al. Alcohol and cancers of the upper aerodigestive tract in men and women. Cancer Epidemiol Biomarkers Prev 1994;3:299–304.

[22] Maier H, Dietz A, Gewelke U, et al. Tobacco and alcohol and the risk of head and neck cancer. Clin Invest 1992;70:320–7.

[23] Blot WJ. Alcohol and cancer. Cancer Res 1992;52:2119s–23.

[24] Schottenfeld D. The etiology and prevention of aerodigestive tract cancers. Adv Exp Med Biol 1992;320:1–19.

[25] Ellwood JM, Pearson JCG, Skippen DH, et al. Alcohol, smoking social and occupational factors in the etiology of cancer of the oral cavity, pharynx and larynx. Int J Cancer 1985;34: 603–12.

[26] Russo D, Purohit V, Foudin L, et al. Workshop on alcohol use and health disparities 2002: a call to arms. Alcohol 2004;32:37–43.

[27] Horowitz AM, Nourjah PA. Factors associated with having oral cancer examinations among US adults 40 years of age or older. J Public Health Dent 1996;56:331–5.

[28] Klassen AC, Juon HS, Alberg AJ, et al. Opportunities for oral cancer screening among older African-American women. Prev Med 2003;37:499–506.

[29] Canto MT, Drury TF, Horowitz AM. Oral cancer examinations among US Hispanics in 1998. J Cancer Educ 2003;18:48–52.

[30] Horowitz AM, Siriphant P, Sheikh A, et al. Perspectives of Maryland dentists on oral cancer. J Am Dent Assoc 2001;132:65–72.

[31] Shavers VL, Harlan LC, Winn D, et al. Racial/ethnic patterns of care for cancer of the oral cavity, pharynx, larynx, sinuses and salivary gland. Cancer Metastasis Rev 2003;22: 25–38.

[32] Arbes SJ Jr, Olshan AF, Caplan DJ, et al. Factors contributing to the poorer survival of black Americans diagnosed with oral cancer (United States). Cancer Causes Control 1999; 10:513–23.

[33] Konski A, Berkey BA, Ang KK, et al. Effect of education level on outcome of patients treated on radiation therapy oncology group protocol 90–03. Cancer 2003;98:1497–503.

[34] Konski AA, Pajak T, Movas B, et al. Socio-demographic variables influence outcome in radiation therapy oncology group head and neck trials. Atlanta (GA): ASTRO; 2004.

[35] Centers for Disease Control and Prevention. Youth risk behavior surveillance—United States, 2001. MMWR Morb Mortal Wkly Rep 2002;51:1–64.

THE MEDICAL CLINICS OF NORTH AMERICA

Med Clin N Am 89 (2005) 1045–1057

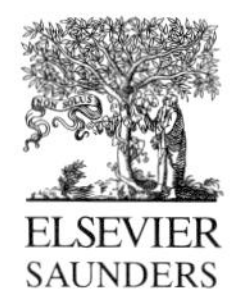

Prognostic Impact of Race and Ethnicity in the Treatment of Colorectal Cancer

Edith P. Mitchell, MD

Division of Medical Oncology, Kimmel Cancer Center, Thomas Jefferson University, Gibbon Building, Suite 4240, Philadelphia, PA 19107, USA

Multiple studies have demonstrated that black patients have a less favorable prognosis and suffer higher death rates from colorectal cancer than whites [1–11]. A review of data from the Surveillance, Epidemiology, and End Results (SEER) Program for the years 1992 to 1997 showed significant disparities in 5-year relative survival rates for all stages of colorectal cancer, with overall survival rates of 60.2% for whites and 51.2% for blacks. This difference in mortality has been attributed to a number of factors, the most important of which was believed to be a more advanced stage of disease at the time of diagnosis [12,13]; however, other possible factors include lack of access to and use of resources in the health care system, presence of comorbid diseases and medical conditions, tolerance of treatment, and tumor responsiveness to treatment [14].

Because there was a similar distribution among cancer stages for whites and blacks during the 1992 to 1997 period, the SEER report further identified a worse 5-year survival for blacks, not only for overall survival but also for each stage: localized, regional, or metastatic disease [13]. There was little information in these reports exploring potential differences in the aggressiveness of tumors or inherent tumor biology. In addition, the specific treatment received by patients was not delineated; therefore, the role of treatment differences as a potential contributing factor in disparities among ethnic groups was not defined.

Although a larger percentage of black patients present with advanced-stage disease, several studies have shown that even after controlling for tumor stage at diagnosis, black patients have worse survival than whites

E-mail address: edith.mitchell@jefferson.edu

doi:10.1016/j.mcna.2005.05.007   *medical.theclinics.com*

[1,13]. Furthermore, after adjusting for other factors such as poverty, socioeconomic conditions, and treatment differences, there was still no clear explanation for survival differences or outcomes. Because most studies incorporated an admixture of proximal, transverse, and distal colon tumors, specified outcomes for rectal cancer as a single entity were not delineated.

After more than 40 years of 5-fluorouracil (5-FU)–based therapy, the introduction of new agents such as irinotecan, oxaliplatin, and capecitabine in the past decade has revolutionized the treatment of colorectal cancer. Although 5-FU remains an important part of most regimens, irinotecan and oxaliplatin are now essential components of front-line therapy. The development of new agents such as bevacizumab, cetuximab, and other targeted therapies currently under investigation, suggest that significant progress in colorectal cancer management will continue. It is therefore particularly important that clinical trials include a wide variety of patients and that patients in populations for whom disparities indicate higher death rates avail themselves of new research developments.

First-line therapy

In the mid-1980s, the recognition that therapy with 5-FU could be enhanced with leucovorin (LV) was an important development in colorectal cancer treatment. A meta-analysis of 18 trials that recently compared the effects of 5-FU to those of 5-FU/LV demonstrated that 5-FU/LV was associated with significantly greater response rates (23% versus 12%) and 1-year survival rates (48% versus 43%) [15].

Another important development was the recognition that chemotherapy with 5-FU could be effectively delivered in multiple regimens. These regimens include the methods of continuous infusions, combinations of bolus doses with continuous infusions, and high-dose infusions administered with folinic acid. A meta-analysis of six trials that compared the efficacy of these regimens reported that continuous infusions of 5-FU resulted in greater response rates, greater survival, and less neutropenia compared with bolus 5-FU [16]. Continuous infusions, however, were associated with a greater incidence of hand-foot syndrome.

In 1996, irinotecan, a novel topoisomerase I inhibitor, was approved by the Food and Drug Administration (FDA) as an important new treatment option for colorectal cancer. Studies of its efficacy as a first-line single-agent therapy for advanced colorectal cancer consistently reported response rates of 20% to 30%, with a mean survival of about 12 months [17–19], and investigators soon recognized the benefit of combining irinotecan with 5-FU/LV. In a phase III United States trial of irinotecan, 5-FU/LV, and irinotecan in combination with 5-FU/LV (IFL) in previously untreated patients who had metastatic colorectal cancer, the IFL group experienced a greater response rate, a greater time to disease progression, and an improvement in overall survival compared with treatment with 5-FU/LV alone [20]. A similar study in Europe reported comparable results [21]. In fact, almost twice as many patients in the European trial responded to IFL compared with 5-FU/LV (41% versus 23%). One-year survival was also significantly greater with IFL compared with 5-FU/LV (69% versus 59%). In this first-line study, IFL significantly improved objective response rates, increased time to disease progression, and prolonged survival compared with 5-FU/LV alone. The FDA approved IFL in March 2000 as first-line therapy for advanced colorectal cancer as a result of these studies.

The next agent that was approved for colorectal cancer treatment was capecitabine, an oral fluoropyrimidine, which was designed to mimic a continuous infusion of 5-FU. After ingestion, capecitabine is absorbed from the gastrointestinal tract and, through a series of metabolic reactions, converted to the active drug 5-FU [22]. Capecitabine is a more convenient treatment than 5-FU and may confer a less severe side-effect profile. Initially, it demonstrated activity as single-agent therapy and in combination with irinotecan and oxaliplatin. In a randomized clinical trial comparing capecitabine to 5-FU/LV in patients who had metastatic disease, capecitabine was associated with a significantly higher objective response rate; however, no differences in survival were noted [23]. One major advantage of capecitabine noted in this trial was a better side-effect profile, with significantly less diarrhea, stomatitis, nausea, alopecia, and neutropenia in the capecitabine group compared with the 5-FU/LV group.

Oxaliplatin, a third-generation platinum compound, was approved by the FDA in 2002 as a second-line treatment in combination with 5-FU/LV for patients whose disease has progressed after IFL. In a phase III trial of infusional 5-FU/LV with or without oxaliplatin, infused 5-FU/LV/ oxaliplatin (FOLFOX; for a description of FOLFOX regimens see Fig. 1 [24]) was associated with a significantly greater response rate compared with 5-FU/LV (49% versus 22%) [25]. The median survival time was similar between groups (15.9 versus 14.7 months).

In 2004, the FDA approved oxaliplatin in combination with infusional 5-FU/LV for first-line therapy for metastatic cancer of the colon and rectum, based on results of the National Cancer Institute N9741 trial [26],

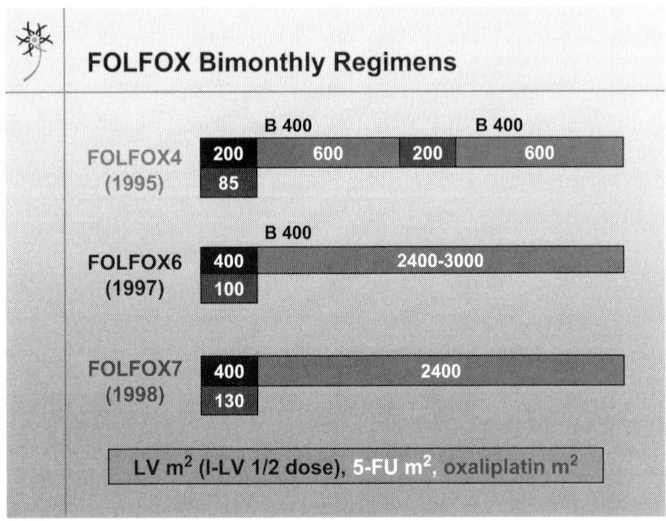

Fig. 1. FOLFOX4, FOLFOX6, and FOLFOX7 regimens.

which was the first study to evaluate the combination of irinotecan/ oxaliplatin. In this study, FOLFOX (with 5-FU infusion) was compared with IFL (with bolus 5-FU) and to irinotecan/oxaliplatin. FOLFOX was associated with a greater rate of response, median time to progression, and overall survival compared with either of the other treatments. A significant difference in favor of FOLFOX was noted in terms of its toxicity profile. Only the incidence of paresthesia was significantly greater with FOLFOX compared with the other therapies. The investigators noted, however, that this study was not designed to identify the relative independent contributions of the agents tested (ie, oxaliplatin versus irinotecan or infused versus bolus 5-FU). Phase III protocols comparing irinotecan with oxaliplatin (both arms using infused 5-FU/LV) are currently being initiated through the National Cancer Institute.

Comparisons of irinotecan/infused 5-FU/LV (FOLFIRI) and FOLFOX have been investigated by Tournigand and colleagues [27] in an effort to determine optimal sequencing of irinotecan and oxaliplatin. In this phase III study of first-line therapy with FOLFIRI (Table 1) or FOLFOX6, patients received FOLFIRI followed by FOLFOX6 at progression, or FOLFOX6 followed by FOLFIRI at progression. Because the median time to progression and median overall survival were similar between groups, the investigators concluded that the two treatments as a first-line agent were equivalent in efficacy (Table 2). Grade 3/4 toxicities were different in the two first-line arms: gastrointestinal toxicities, except diarrhea, were more

Table 1
Tournigand phase III trial of first-line FOLFIRI/FOLFOX6

Detail	Arm A		Arm B		
	FOLFIRI	FOLFOX	FOLFOX	FOLFIRI	*P* value
Overall response risk	56[a]	15	54[a]	4	0.68
Median total therapy	14.4	—	—	11.5	0.65
Median overall survival	20.4	—	—	21.5	0.9
Liver resections	7.3	—	—	18.9	

[a] First-line overall response rate.

Data from Tournigand C, Louvet C, Quinaux E, et al. FOLFIRI followed by FOLFOX followed by FOLFIRI in metastatic colorectal cancer (MCRC): final results of a phase III study [abstract 494]. Proc Am Soc Clin Oncol 2001;21.

significant in the FOLFIRI arm, and hematologic and neurotoxicities were more severe in the FOLFOX6 arm. Because both agents demonstrated equal efficacy as first-line therapy, Douillard [28] suggested that secondary endpoints such as toxicity, second-line efficacy, and compliance to treatment favor FOLFIRI as first-line therapy.

Because capecitabine is considered to be equivalent to 5-FU in efficacy, combinations of capecitabine and irinotecan or oxaliplatin have been evaluated. The response rates and time to disease progression with irinotecan/capecitabine and oxaliplatin/capecitabine have been shown to be similar to those observed with irinotecan or oxaliplatin in combination with 5-FU [29,30]. In a study that compared the efficacy of irinotecan/capecitabine to that of oxaliplatin/capecitabine, investigators reported similar response rates (38% with irinotecan and 42% with oxaliplatin) and overall survival (15.8 months in both groups) in both treatment arms [31]. These results and the safety of these combinations were validated in a study of these combinations as second-line therapy, presented at the 2004 American Society of Clinical Oncology Annual Meeting [32].

Table 2
Median overall survival correlates with availability of all three effective drugs

First author, year [Ref.]	Patients with 3 drugs (%)	Overall survival (mo)
Saltz, 2000 [20]	5	14.8
Douillard, 2000 [21]	16	17.4
De Gramont, 2000 [25]	29	16.2
Giacchetti, 2000 [47]	60	19.4
Tournigand, 2001 [24]	68	21.0
Goldberg, 2004 [26]	70	19.5
Grothey, 2002 [48]	75	21.4

Preliminary results of a phase I/II study of first-line treatment with oxaliplatin, irinotecan, 5-FU, and LV have been promising [33]. In this study, investigators reported a response rate of 78%, a much higher rate than is typically observed with current therapeutic combinations.

In summary, in first-line treatment of colorectal cancer, when the fluoropyrimidine is held constant with a 5-FU regimen or capecitabine, the addition of either oxaliplatin or irinotecan regimens result in similar activity. The side-effect profiles, however, are different. Typical toxicities observed with FOLFIRI are related to the gastrointestinal tract, whereas FOLFOX is associated with neurotoxicities.

Combination therapy using targeted agents

Recent progress in the management of colorectal cancer has involved the development and approval of two targeted agents (bevacizumab and cetuximab) and the investigational agent PTK787/ZK 222,584 (PTK/ZK). The most active areas of investigation are their efficacy, safety, and optimal usage in combination with cytotoxic therapy.

One of the major processes that occurs when tumors increase in size from a small tumor (< 2 mm) to a large, visible tumor is the angiogenic switch. The angiogenic switch occurs after events that result in the upregulation of angiogenic factors that stimulate angiogenesis, causing rapid tumor growth and promoting metastasis [34]. One central mediator of angiogenesis is vascular endothelial growth factor, which is overexpressed in many tumor types. Vascular endothelial growth factor rapidly stimulates endothelial cell functions, increases vascular permeability and the survival of immature vasculature, promotes lymphangiogenesis, and may inhibit the tumoral immune response.

Bevacizumab, a monoclonal antibody against vascular endothelial growth factor, has shown considerable promise in the treatment of colorectal cancer. In 2004, the FDA approved the use of bevacizumab in combination with intravenous 5-FU–based chemotherapy for first-line treatment of metastatic colon or rectal cancer. In a phase II trial of 5-FU/LV with and without bevacizumab in metastatic colorectal cancer, response rates, time to progression, and median survival were significantly greater with the addition of low-dose bevacizumab (5 mg/kg every 2 weeks) [35]. A pivotal phase III trial of first-line bolus IFL plus bevacizumab also showed significant increases in median survival, progression-free survival, response rates, and duration of response with IFL plus bevacizumab compared with IFL alone [36]. The median duration of survival was 20.3 months in the group given IFL plus bevacizumab compared with 15.6 months in the control arm (IFL plus placebo). A subgroup of patients in this study received second-line treatment with oxaliplatin. In this group, median overall survival was 25.1 months for patients receiving IFL plus bevacizumab and 22.2 months in the group given IFL plus placebo.

The primary side effect associated with IFL plus bevacizumab was hypertension, which was easily managed with standard oral antihypertensives such as calcium channel blockers, angiotensin-converting enzyme inhibitors, or diuretics. A new potential adverse event was gastrointestinal perforation, although this was uncommon and had variable clinical presentation. Ongoing studies are addressing the role of oxaliplatin/bevacizumab combinations; however, there are not yet sufficient long-term data to allow evaluation of the efficacy of such combinations [36].

An antiangiogenic agent under investigation is PTK/ZK, an oral compound that is a potent and relatively selective inhibitor of the vascular endothelial growth factor receptor tyrosine kinases. Ongoing studies are evaluating its efficacy in combination with irinotecan- and oxaliplatin-based therapy. MRI studies have shown that PTK/ZK administration inhibits tumor vascular enhancement as early as one day after its administration [37].

Another active area of investigation is the role of the epidermal growth factor receptor (EGFR) in cancer. This receptor has been shown to regulate tumor cell division, repair, survival, and metastasis [38]. Binding of ligands to the receptor triggers an intracellular signaling cascade. The inhibition of EGFR may affect the growth or the progression of EGFR-expressing tumors such as colorectal cancer. Epidermal growth factor receptor levels are correlated with poor prognosis, decreased survival, and increased metastasis.

There are two primary types of anti-EGFR therapies: monoclonal antibodies, which bind to the ligand-binding domain, preventing the initiation of intracellular signaling; and tyrosine kinase inhibitors, which inhibit the activity of the EGFR pathway. Cetuximab is a monoclonal antibody to EGFR that prevents ligands from binding to the receptor and that downregulates EGFR expression, tyrosine kinase phosphorylation, and signal transduction.

The efficacy of cetuximab in combination with irinotecan has been evaluated in a study of patients refractory to 5-FU/irinotecan whose tumors are EGFR positive [39]. The combination was associated with a median survival of 9 months and was equally efficacious in patients who had mild, moderate, or strong EGFR expression. Based on this study, the FDA approved cetuximab as a single agent or in combination with irinotecan as second-line therapy to treat EGFR-expressing metastatic colorectal cancer.

Second-line therapy

Patients with metastatic colorectal cancer who have progressed on first-line therapy have numerous options. The choice of second-line therapy is based primarily on which regimen the patient received upfront: 5-FU/LV or single-agent capecitabine; IFL or FOLFIRI, or FOLFOX. Other considerations include the quality and duration of response to first-line treatment, the toxicities experienced, and the current condition and function of the patient.

Irinotecan and oxaliplatin were originally approved as second-line therapies for patients whose disease had progressed after standard therapy. In two registration trials of irinotecan, irinotecan was compared with best supportive care and a continuos infusion of 5-FU in patients whose cancers had progressed after treatment with bolus 5-FU/LV [19,40]. In both trials, the mean survival time and the 1-year survival rate for patients on irinotecan were significantly greater than those observed with best supportive care and infusion of 5-FU.

In a recent registration trial of FOLFOX4 compared with infusional 5-FU/LV and oxaliplatin alone in patients who had colorectal cancer progression after treatment with IFL, Rothenberg and colleagues [40] reported that response rates, time to disease progression, overall survival, and relief from tumor-related symptoms was significantly greater with FOLFOX than with infusional 5-FU/LV or oxaliplatin alone. In fact, when median overall survival was compared with the percentage of patients who received three drugs (irinotecan, oxaliplatin, and 5-FU or capecitabine) in recent studies of metastatic colorectal cancer, overall survival increased with the percentage of patients who received all three agents.

Patients whose tumors express EGFR have another option of receiving cetuximab as a single agent or in combination with irinotecan following irinotecan failure, based on the results of the study by Cunningham and colleagues [39] described previously (see "Combination therapy using targeted agents"). An ongoing phase III trial (CA225-006) is comparing cetuximab/irinotecan with irinotecan alone following progression on an oxaliplatin-based regimen. The use of bevacizumab as salvage therapy is still under active investigation.

Treatment of liver-limited metastases

Nearly half of patients who have colorectal cancer will develop liver metastases during the course of their disease [41]. In one study of the impact of preoperative chemotherapy on patient outcome in patients who had liver-limited metastatic disease, 58% of patients who responded to chemotherapy and 45% of patients whose disease was stable were alive after 3 years [42]. In contrast, none of the 28 patients whose disease progressed on chemotherapy was living 3 years later. Therefore, response to chemotherapy was predictive of survival benefit in patients who had multiple hepatic lesions undergoing liver resection.

In another recent trial of 42 patients whose liver metastases were determined to be nonoptimally resectable for surgical evaluation, 62% of patients responded to FOLFOX therapy [43]. Patients who then underwent resection survived for a median duration of 31.4 months. Because the mean survival in patients who do not receive surgery is 21 months, surgery may enhance survival in patients who respond to chemotherapy and whose metastases are limited to the liver.

Adjuvant therapy

Irinotecan, oxaliplatin, and 5-FU/LV may aid in the treatment of high-risk patients who have resected stage II and III cancers. In a pooled analysis of the impact of adjuvant therapy for colorectal cancer, Gill and colleagues [44] reported that the use of 5-FU/LV or 5-FU/levamisole after surgery was associated with a 35% reduction in the risk of disease recurrence compared with no treatment. The 5-year disease-free survival rates were 69% with adjuvant therapy and 59% without therapy. In addition, model-derived estimates of 5-year disease-free survival showed that the beneficial effect of adjuvant therapy (over surgery alone) rose with increasing T stage and number of involved nodes.

The impact of FOLFOX in patients after resection of stage II or III colorectal cancer has also been compared with that of infusional 5-FU/LV in a randomized clinical trial. At 3 years, patients on FOLFOX experienced a 23% reduction in the risk of disease progression compared with infusional 5-FU/LV [25]. This benefit was observed in patients who had stage II and stage III disease. Upcoming adjuvant studies will evaluate the addition of bevacizumab to chemotherapy and another study will compare the use of FOLFOX, FOLFIRI, and the sequential use of FOLFOX followed by FOLFIRI [45].

Several trials have investigated the impact of chemotherapy and con-comitant irradiation in locally advanced or recurrent adenocarcinoma of the rectum. A phase I/II trial of the effects of irinotecan/5-FU found that 100% of patients achieved a complete (57%) or partial (43%) response [46]. At the time of surgery, 25% of patients achieved a complete pathologic response, which is considerably greater than the 12% to 15% response rates usually observed with 5-FU and concomitant irradiation.

Summary

Numerous advances in the treatment of patients who have metastatic disease have improved colorectal cancer management, including new chemotherapeutic agents and combinations and targeted agents that modulate the efficacy of chemotherapy. Recent advances in the administration of irinotecan and oxaliplatin, in combination with 5-FU/LV, plus the addition of targeted agents bevacizumab and cetuximab have afforded steady increases in response rates and survival. Ongoing studies are evaluating the optimal sequencing and combinations of the agents described and the efficacy of new combinations in metastatic and adjuvant settings. Because the number of African-American patients in most clinical trials in colorectal cancer has been low, it is imperative that method increase participation so that new research developments reach all segments of the population.

References

[1] Ries LA, Eisner MP, Kosary CL, et al. SEER Cancer Statistics Review, 1973–1998. Bethesda (MD): National Cancer Institute; 2001.

[2] Parker SL, Davis KJ, Wingo PA, et al. Cancer statistics by race and ethnicity [abstract]. CA Cancer J Clin 1998;48:31–48.

[3] Axtel LM, Myers MH. Contrasts in survival of black and white cancer patients, 1960–1973. J Natl Cancer Inst 1978;60:1209–15.

[4] Young JL, Ries LG, Pollack ES. Cancer patient survival among ethnic groups in the United States. J Natl Cancer Inst 1984;3:341–52.

[5] Wingo PA, Ries LA, Parker SL, et al. Long-term cancer patient survival in the United States [abstract]. Cancer Epidemiol Biomarkers Prev 1998;7:271–82.

[6] Chen VW, Fenoglio-Preiser CM, Wu Xc, et al. Aggressiveness of colon carcionoma in blacks and whites. National Cancer Institute Black/White Cancer Survival Study Group [abstract]. Cancer Epidemiol Biomarkers Prev 1997;6:1087–93.

[7] Demers RY, Serverson RK, Schottenfeld D, et al. Incidence of colorectal adenocarcinoma by anatomic subsite. An epidemiologic study of time trends and racial differences in the Detroit, Michigan area. Cancer 1997;79:441–7.

[8] Beart RW, Steele GD Jr, Menck HR, et al. Management and survival of patients with adenocarcinoma of the colon and rectum: a national survey of the Commission on Cancer. J Am Coll Surg 1995;181:225–36.

[9] Daya H, Polissar L, Yang CT, et al. Race, socioeconomic status, and other prognostic factors for survival from colorectal cancer. J Chronic Dis 1987;40:857–64.

[10] Cooper GS, Yuan Z, Rimm AA. Racial disparity in the incidence and case-fatality of colorectal cancer: analysis of 329 United States counties [abstract]. Cancer Epidemiol Biomarkers Prev 1997;6:283–95.

[11] Mayberry RM, Coates RJ, Hill HA, et al. Determinants of black/white differences in colon cancer survival [abstract]. J Natl Cancer Instit 1995;87:1686–93.

[12] Dignam JJ, Ye Y, Colangelo L, et al. Prognosis after rectal cancer in blacks and whites participating in adjuvant therapy randomized trials. J Clin Oncol 2003;21(3):413–20.

[13] Ries LA, Wingo PA, Miller DS, et al. The annual report to the nation on the status of cancer, 1973–1997, with a special section on colorectal cancer. Cancer 2000;88: 2398–424.

[14] McCollum AD, Catalano PJ, Haller DB, et al. Outcomes and toxicity in African-American and Caucasian patients in a randomized adjuvant chemotherapy trial for colon cancer [abstract]. J Natl Cancer Inst 2002;94:1160–7.

[15] Piedbois P, Michiels S. Survival benefit of 5FU/LV over 5FU bolus in patients with advanced colorectal cancer: an updated meta-analysis based on 2,751 patients [abstract 1180]. Proc Am Soc Clin Oncol 2003;22:294.

[16] Meta-Analysis Group in Cancer. Efficacy of intravenous continuous infusion of fluorouacil compared with bolus administration in advanced colorectal cancer. J Clin Oncol 1998;16: 301–8.

[17] Conti JA, Kemeny NE, Saltz LB, et al. Irinotecan is an active agent in untreated patients with metastatic colorectal cancer. J Clin Oncol 1996;14:709–15.

[18] Pitot HC, Wender DB, O'Connell MJ, et al. Phase II trial of irinotecan in patients with metastatic colorectal carcinoma. J Clin Oncol 1997;15:2910–9.

[19] Rougier P, Bugat R, Douillard JY, et al. Phase II study of irinotecan in the treatment of advanced colorectal cancer in chemotherapy-naive patients and patients pretreated with fluorouracil-based chemotherapy. J Clin Oncol 1997;15:251–60.

[20] Saltz LB, Cox JV, Blanke C, et al. Irinotecan plus fluorouracil and leucovorin for metastatic colorectal cancer. Irinotecan Study Group. N Engl J Med 2000;343:905–14.

[21] Douillard JY, Cunningham D, Roth AD, et al. Irinotecan combined with fluorouracil compared with fluorouracil along as first line treatment for metastatic colorectal cancer: a multicentre randomized trial. Lancet 2000;355:1041–7.

[22] Roche Laboratories, Inc. Xeloda complete product information. Nutley (NJ): Roche Laboratories; 2003.

[23] Hoff PM, Ansari R, Batist G, et al. Comparison of oral capecitabine versus intravenous fluorouracil plus leucovorin as fist line treatment in 605 patients with metastatic colorectal cancer: results of a randomized phase III study. J Clin Oncol 2001;19:2282–92.

[24] Tournigand C, Louvet C, Puinaux E, et al. FOLFIRI followed by FOLFOX versus FOLFOX followed by FOLFIRI in metastatic colorectal cancer (MCRC): final results of a phase III study [abstract 494]. Proc Am Soc Clin Oncol 2001;21.

[25] de Gramont A, Figer A, Seymour M, et al. Leucovorin and fluorouracil with or without oxaliplatin as firstline treatment in advanced colorectal cancer. J Clin Oncol 2000;18: 2938–47.

[26] Goldberg R, Sargent DJ, Morton RF, et al. A randomized controlled trial of fluorouracil plus leucovorin, irinotecan, and oxaliplatin combinations in patients with previously untreated metastatic colorectal cancer. J Clin Oncol 2004;22:23–30.

[27] Tournigand C, Andre T, Achille E, et al. FOLFIRI followed by FOLFOX6 or the reverse sequence in advanced colorectal cancer: a randomized GERCOR study. J Clin Oncol 2004; 22:229–37.

[28] Douillard JY. The new generation of CRC therapy: extending survival and the continuum of care [abstract]. Academy for Healthcare Education's The GI Cancer Challenge: Establishing Treatment Strategies Within the Evolving Paradigm Symposium conducted at the American Society of Clinical Oncology 40th Annual Meeting. New Orleans, Louisiana, June 5–8, 2004.

[29] Van Cutsem E, Twelves C, Taberno J, et al. XELOX: mature results of a multinational, phase II trial of capecitabine plus oxaliplatin, an effective 1st line option for patients with

metastatic colorectal cancer [abstract]. Proc Am Soc Clin Oncol 2003;22:255 [Abstract 1023.].

[30] Patt YZ, Lin E, Leibmann J, et al. Capecitabine plus irinotecan for chemotherapy-naïve patients with metastatic colorectal cancer (MCRC): US multicenter phase II trial [abstract]. Proc Am Soc Clin Oncol 2003;22:281 [Abstract 1130.].

[31] Grothey A, Jordan K, Kellner O, et al. Randomized phase II trial of capecitabine plus irinotecan (CapIri) vs capecitabine plus oxaliplatin. (CapOx) as first line therapy of advanced colorectal cancer [abstract 1022]. Proc Am Soc Clin Oncol 2003;22:255.

[32] Grothey A, Jordan K, Kellner O, et al. Capecitabine/irinotecan (CapeIri) and capecitabine/oxaliplatin (CapeOx) are active second line protocols in patients with advanced colorectal cancer (ACRC) after failure of first line combination therapy: results of a randomized phase II study [abstract 3534]. Proc Am Soc Clin Oncol 2004;23:254.

[33] Roth AD, Seium Y, Ruhstaller T, et al. Oxaliplatin combined with irinotecan (CPT-11) and 5FU/leucovorin in metastatic colorectal cancer: a phase I–II study [abstract 570]. Proc Am Soc Clin Oncol 2002;21:143a.

[34] Carmeliet P, Jain RK. Angiogenesis in cancer and other diseases. Nature 2000;407:249–57.

[35] Kabbinavar F, Hurwitz HI, Fehrenbacher L, et al. Phase II, randomized trial comparing bevacizumab plus fluorouracil (FU)/leucovorin (LV) with FU/LV alone in patient with metastatic colorectal cancer. J Clin Oncol 2003;21:60–5.

[36] Hurwitz H, Fehrenbacher L, Novotny W, et al. Bevacizumab plus irinotecan, fluorouracil, and leucovorin for metastatic colorectal cancer. N Engl J Med 2004;350:2335–42.

[37] Morgan B, Thomas AL, Drevs J, et al. Dynamic contrast-enhanced magnetic resonance imaging as a biomarker for the pharmacological response of PTK787/ZK 222584, an inhibitor of the vascular endothelial growth factor receptor tyrosine kinases, in patients with advanced colorectal cancer and liver metastases: results from two phase I studies. J Clin Oncol 2003;21:3955–64.

[38] Harari PM, Huang SM. Modulation of molecular targets to enhance radiation. Clin Cancer Res 2000;6:323–5.

[39] Cunningham D, Humblet Y, Siena S, et al. Cetuximab (C225) alone or in combination with irinotecan (CPT-11) in patients with epidermal growth factor receptor (EGFR)-positive, irinotecan refractory metastastatic colorectal cancer [abstract 1012]. Proc Am Soc Clin Oncol 2003;22:252.

[40] Cunningham D, Pyrhonen S, James RD, et al. Randomised trial of irinotecan plus supportive care versus supportive care alone after fluorouracil failure for patients with metastatic colorectal cancer. Lancet 1998;352:1413–8.

[41] Rothenberg ML, Oza AM, Burger B, et al. Final results of a phase III trial of 5-FU/leucovorin versus oxaliplatin versus the combination in patients with metastatic colorectal cancer following irinotecan, 5-FU, and leucovorin [abstract 1011]. Proc Am Soc Clin Oncol 2003;22:252.

[42] Yoon SS, Tanabe KK. Surgical treatment and other regional treatments for colorectal cancer liver metastases. Oncologist 1999;4:197–208.

[43] Adam R, Pascal G, Castaing D, et al. Liver resection for multiple colorectal metastases: Influence of preoperative chemotherapy [abstract 1188]. Proc Am Soc Clin Oncol 2003;22:296.

[44] Alberts SR, Donohue JH, Mahoney MR, et al. Liver resection after 5-fluorouracil, leucovorin and oxaliplatin for patients with metastatic colorectal cancer limited to the liver: a North Central Cancer Treatment Group (NCCTG) phase II study [abstract 1053]. Proc Am Soc Clin Oncol 2003;22:263.

[45] Gill S, Loprinzi CL, Sargent DJ, et al. Pooled analysis of fluorouracil-based adjuvant therapy for stage II and III colon cancer: who benefits and by how much? J Clin Oncol 2004; 22:1797–806.

[46] O'Connell MJ. Current status of adjuvant therapy for colorectal cancer. Oncology 2004;18: 751–5.

[47] Giacchetti. 2000.

[48] Grothey. 2002.

Med Clin N Am 89 (2005) 1059

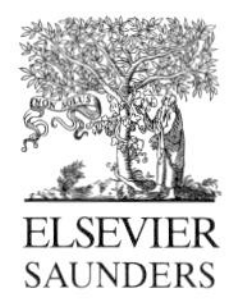

THE MEDICAL CLINICS OF NORTH AMERICA

Erratum

Rheumatic Diseases in Minority Populations

Gail S. Kerr, MD, FRCP(Edin)[a,b,c],
J. Steuart Richards, MD[a,b], E. Nigel Harris, MD, PhD[d]

[a]*Rheumatology Section, Veterans Affairs Medical Center, 50 Irving Street,
NW, Washington, DC 20422, USA*
[b]*Department of Medicine, Georgetown University, Washington, DC, USA*
[c]*Department of Medicine, Howard University Hospitals, Washington, DC, USA*
[d]*University of the West Indies, Vice Chancellery, Mona, Kingston 7, Jamaica, West Indies*

This article originally published in the *Medical Clinics of North America*, Volume 89, Issue 4, pages 829–868. The authors would like to acknowledge the following contributions:

Acknowledgments

The authors acknowledge the contributions of their research assistants, Shari Boyce and Adassa Richardson, and Mary Rust for her assistance in preparing the manuscript.

doi:10.1016/j.mcna.2005.08.009

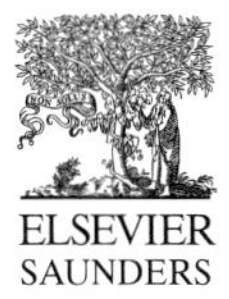

ELSEVIER
SAUNDERS

Med Clin N Am 89 (2005) 1061–1066

THE MEDICAL
CLINICS
OF NORTH AMERICA

Index

Note: Page numbers of article titles are in **boldface** type.

A

Acarbose, for diabetes mellitus, 963–964

Acetohexamide, for diabetes mellitus, 964

Acute coronary syndromes, in African Americans, 987–991

Adherence issues
in coronary heart disease, 993–994
in diabetes mellitus, 957

Aerodigestive tract cancer, in minorities, **1033–1043**
diagnosis of, 1038–1040
epidemiology of, 1033–1035
mortality in, 1033–1034, 1040–1041
risk factors for, 1035–1038
treatment of, 1040–1041

African Americans
aerodigestive tract cancer in, **1033–1043**
diagnosis of, 1038–1040
epidemiology of, 1033–1035
mortality in, 1033–1034, 1040–1041
risk factors for, 1035–1038
treatment of, 1040–1041
colorectal cancer in, prognosis of, **1045–1057**
with combination therapy, 1049–1050
with first-line therapy, 1046–1049
with liver-limited metastases, 1051–1052
with second-line therapy, 1050–1051
coronary heart disease in, **977–1001**
acute coronary syndromes in, 987–991
clinical spectrum of, 977
diagnosis of, 991
historical perspective of, 978–980
pathophysiology of, 986–987
prevention of, 992–994
risk factors for, 980–985, 991
diabetes mellitus in. *See* Diabetes mellitus, type 2, in minorities.

emergency surgical care for, **945–948**
hypertension in, **921–933**
epidemiology of, 922–923
pathophysiology of, 923–926
psychosocial issues in, 926–927
renal transplantation and, 1005–1006
salt-sensitive, 924
treatment of, 927–930
kidney transplantation in, **1003–1031**
barriers to, 1006–1012
candidates for, 1004–1006
outcomes of, 1012–1022
remedies for disparities in, 1022–1025
women's reproductive health issues in, **935–943**
cervical cancer, 940–941
endometrial cancer, 940
infertility, 935–937
maternal mortality, 937
ovarian cancer, 939–940
prenatal care, 938–939
preterm births, 937–938

African-American Study of Kidney Disease and Hypertension trial, 930

Alcohol use, aerodigestive tract cancer and, 1038

ALLHAT (Antihypertensive and Lipid-Lowering Treatment to Prevent Heart Attacks), in African Americans, 929–930

Alpha-blockers, for hypertension, 927

Alpha-glucosidase inhibitors, for diabetes mellitus, 963–964

American Indians. *See* Native Americans.

Amputation, in diabetes mellitus, in minorities, 950

Angina, in African Americans, 987–991

Angiotensin II, elevated, in hypertension, 923–924

Changing Your Address?

Make sure your subscription changes too! When you notify us of your new address, you can help make our job easier by including an exact copy of your Clinics label number with your old address (see illustration below.) This number identifies you to our computer system and will speed the processing of your address change. Please be sure this label number accompanies your old address and your corrected address—you can send an old Clinics label with your number on it or just copy it exactly and send it to the address listed below.

We appreciate your help in our attempt to give you continuous coverage. Thank you.

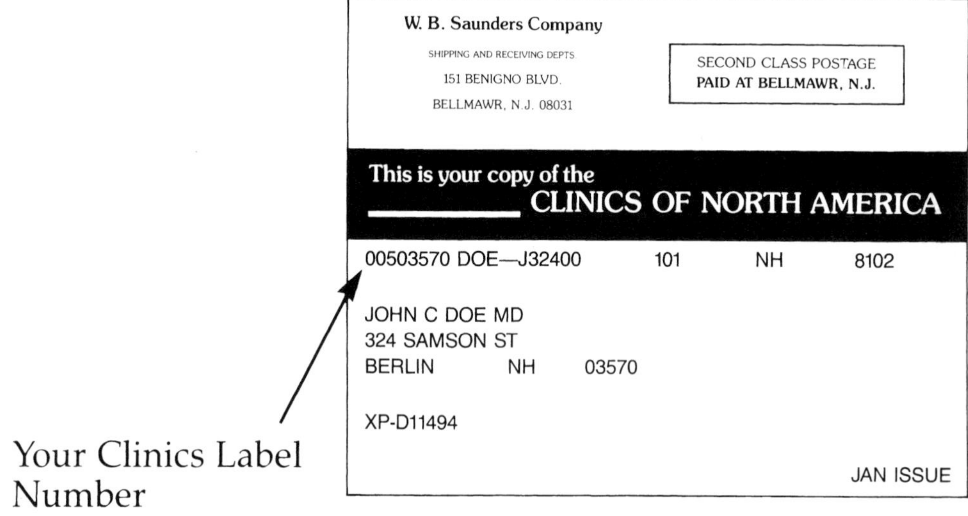

Your Clinics Label Number

Copy it exactly or send your label along with your address to:
W.B. Saunders Company, Customer Service
Orlando, FL 32887-4800
Call Toll Free 1-800-654-2452

Please allow four to six weeks for delivery of new subscriptions and for processing address changes.